HOW TO EAT AND LIVE LONGER

REGINALD J. EADIE, MD

A SPIRITUALLY INSPIRED GUIDE TO DIRECT
AFRICAN-AMERICANS INTO A LIFE OF PEACE,
GOOD HEALTH AND LONGEVITY

Introducing
THE EAT RIGHT-SUNLIGHT THEORY™

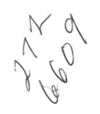

"My people perish because of the lack of knowledge"

Disclaimer

The information, guidance and recommendations contained in this book are based upon the research, as well as personal and professional experiences of the author. It is a source of information only. You are advised to consult your healthcare professional before making any changes in your diet, medications, health plans, lifestyle or way of living. This information should by no means be considered a substitute for the advice of your qualified medical professional. The publisher and author are not responsible for any adverse effects or consequences resulting from the use of any of the suggestions, preparations or procedures discussed in this book. All efforts have been made to ensure the accuracy of the information contained in this book as of the date of publication.

All of the recommendations and procedures contained herein are made without guarantee on the part of the author or the publisher, their agents, or employees. The author and publisher expressly disclaim all liability in connection with the use of this information.

Cover Photo by Stephanie Yelder-Stovall
Cover design by Maurice Nash, ALAN web Solutions LLC
www.alanwebsolutions.com

Printed in the United States
ISBN: 978-1-4276-0791-1

Dedication

My life belongs to my Heavenly Father, who is: the creator of all, the King of Kings, the Lord of Lords, the Master of my fate, the Captain of my soul and the One who holds dominion over all. So it is to Him that I dedicate this book and, I thank you, Father.

I must also recognize the mothers of creation within my life. To my great-grandmothers: Isabella, Rosa, Mary and Ida Belle; my grandmothers: Lillie Mae and Janie; my beautiful mother: Eartha; my gifted sister: Tanya; my God daughter: Doja; and the most precious gifts God could ever give me, my daughters: Brooklyn and Chavis; and their wonder mother: Tauna.

Acknowledgements

It was certainly a pleasure working with those that encouraged me to write a book that the African-American community could use as a supplement in their quest to eat and live longer. Without my African ancestors, my African-American ancestors and the African-American community, we wouldn't have a measuring rod to appreciate where we went wrong (with our eating) and what it is doing to us.

To the Xi Psi & Tau Kappa Kappa chapters of Omega Psi Phi, I am grateful for you all being my listening board, reading my many e-mails on healthy living and being my gateway to the community. To the members of the chapter that lost weight by simply eliminating pork and beef from their diet, stay strong and keep up the good work. To Jamie Brooks, our minister of exercise, we appreciate your perseverance and patience. Uncle Steve Frails, thank you for taking me along with you down the never ending road to knowledge seeking.

To the many clergy men and women that allowed me to speak to their congregations, I appreciate you all for allowing me to exercise my passion and share my findings to the children of God. We all realize that our bodies are temples and that they belong to God and not ourselves.

My friends and colleagues at the Veteran's Administration Hospital , Sinai-Grace Hospital and Crittenton Medical Center who have been waiting patiently to see what Dr. Eadie had to say "this time" about eating to live longer; there is much more to come! My reading those many books in between shifts is what got me to this point. Your patience will forever be remembered and I hope that it will be there for me in the near future. Thanks Lisa Marie Butler for your brilliance, kindness and help.

My family has been just that to me; a family. They have provided that unspoken yet abundant support and love that every revolutionary needs. God surrounded me with perfect grandparents, parents, brothers, sisters, aunts, uncles, cousins, nieces and nephews. May God continue to bless the seeds of Hilliard Eadie and John Johnson. And may their seeds maintain a commitment to God, health and each other.

Table of Contents

Introduction

And the Lord God commanded the man, saying, "Of every tree of the garden you may freely eat; but of the tree of the knowledge of good and evil you shall not eat, for in the day that you eat of it you shall surely die." (Genesis 2:16-17, Holy Bible)

According to the Bible, our perfect God made man after His own image, which in the beginning made man Godly, or humanly perfect. The demise of man began after he committed his very first sin...eating a forbidden food. God warned man that if he ate what he was advised not to, he would surely die. In my opinion, God the omnipotent, had man's first sin be improper eating for a very profound and prophetic reason. He could have chosen this sin to be stealing, adultery, fornication, idol worship, lying, taking the Lord God's name in vain, dishonoring parents, killing, or some other transgression. Instead, He determined that it would involve the act of eating an ill-advised food substance. He is all knowing. And He knew that food would eventually become an impediment for man.

Just as Adam and Eve ate the wrong things, African-Americans are savoring, desiring and becoming slaves to foods that are destroying them and greatly multiplying their sorrows. Today, it is as if America has become the *Garden of Eden* for African-Americans and the forbidden "fruit" (from the tree of knowledge of good and evil) has become our post-slavery cuisine. This aimless quest to satisfy our taste bud's exposure to a seemingly tantalizing aroma is the very reason why African-Americans die sooner than any other inhabitant in this country and our children are living shorter lives than their parents.

Since our unsolicited arrival onto North American soil, our bodies have been struggling to adapt to this new yet defecting way of life. Some of our interactions with these surroundings (i.e. many of the foods we eat) have presented a mental and physical challenge that influences our genes in such a manner that our organ systems began to malfunction. As a result, we are experiencing health problems unlike any other group of persons in America. Our increase in body weight, caused by an excessive accumulation of fat, is directly related to the mental, physical and genetic disarray that is occurring within our community.

A new science exists and research is taking place that will better support my works and will provide more clarification on how those of African descendent are affected by this new "American" lifestyle. This means that the things that you put into your mouth can change your genetic make-up; hence changing who you are, your state of mind and your wellness. In other words, changing the way you think, the way you act, the way you deal with life situations, your risks for diseases, your life span and cause of death, your children's behavior in school, your child's growth patterns, the onset of your daughter's first menstrual cycle (period), etc. Life then becomes more difficult for us and we find it harder to reach our full potential. Through DNA, we began to take on the characteristics of the plants and animals we eat. We are living proof that the cliché "*you are what you eat*" is true!

Working in both urban and suburban Emergency Departments, I have spent the last ten years caring for African-Americans who suffer from diseases that are not common in rural Africa and that come largely as a result of the way we eat here in America. I realized that my short bedside lectures were ineffective and I grew tired of seeing preventable deaths. Each patient repeatedly reminded me of how common improper eating and obesity has become among African-Americans. It has become the norm for our grandmothers to be a "big momma", for our fathers to have a "beer belly", for our children to be "chubby" and for our daughters to develop early. No one is reminding us that these are all signs of unhealthiness and signals of disease and of early death. Not many concern themselves enough to teach us how what we eat shortens our life span or what we should be eating to live longer.

I first thought to use the church as a means of bringing this to the forefront since the church is the one establishment that, throughout the years, has been a constant source of strength and guidance for African-Americans. I quickly pulled the plug on that thought after bearing in mind that many deacons, choir members, church mothers, ushers and Pastors were at least overweight if not morbidly obese. Proper eating and living a long and prosperous life while doing the will of God couldn't be high on the church's agenda. This isn't being taught within the church and I didn't want to stir up the pot. It is very typical for our churches to provide a Sunday morning spiritual meal for our souls (from the pulpit) and then fill our stomachs with deadly foods immediately following the morning worship service. A typical fund raiser for a church guild would be the selling of dinners after the morning service. The dinners would consist of the very foods that contribute to our sickness and death (e.g. fatty and salty pork, foods high in sugars, fried foods full of saturated and trans-fats, dairy products, etc). I am yet to learn of obese prophets in the Bible, Qur'an or Torah. As a Christian, I asked myself: What would Jesus do? What did Jesus eat? What were we to learn from his acts and teachings of eating and fasting? Wasn't God interested in the "whole"? Could you really do God's will effectively while suffering from debilitating illnesses?

At work, school and in public settings we seem to have a troubled nature. This nature is an unnatural condition for God's people. African-Americans look angry, dissatisfied, uninterested, and not focused. On the other hand, when at cookouts, pot-lucks, restaurants or other food endowed places, the woes of life seem to be forgotten. I noticed how food instantaneously changes our demeanor and how suddenly everyone appears happy. As if the food was a drug satisfying the addicts fix, babies become playful, children well behaved and parents joyous and cheerful. The poet, KRS-1 once claimed that beef (instead of crack cocaine) was the number one drug on the streets (of inner city America) and I believe there is a great amount of truth to his writings. To prove his point, he asked his supporters to stop eating beef. I assume he understood how beef (and the many chemicals within it) affects our genes, makes us gain weight and causes us to display addictive characteristics.

Next, I thought about using the school system as a means of communicating to the masses, but that thought was also short lived. Many teachers, counselors, assistant-principals and principals of African descent also have a problem with their weight. As role models, they have to accept some of the responsibility for the new statistics relating to our problem with childhood obesity. Healthy living, nutrition and exercise must be considered to be just as important as reading, writing and arithmetic.

According to a 2006 CBC News article, "Morbid Obesity in Toddlers linked to lower IQ," allowing our offspring to become obese may interfere with their ability to learn, progress and cope with life.[1] I stayed focused on the fact that African-Americans need to learn how to eat to live instead of living to eat. This way, we can live longer, healthier, and more progressive lives...just as our God intended us to do!

I remembered a book that I read when I attended South Carolina State University years ago. It was authored by the Honorable Elijah Muhammad, and was entitled *How to Eat to Live*. This was a very popular book in the 1960's. For its time, it was an easy read and an excellent guide for African-Americans on proper eating. It did, however, lack scientific support and is difficult to apply today since we now know much more about metabolic function and because science and food have changed greatly since then. As a way to pay homage to Elijah Muhammad for his relentless effort, I titled this book *How to Eat and Live Longer*. From what I have read about Mr. Muhammad, I am sure he would appreciate me finishing his plate. After all, truth and knowledge should be our only smorgasbord. Thank you Mr. Muhammad.

Contrary to the belief of many scholars, scientists, physicians and the insurance industry, *obesity is a disease*. It is no less a disease than diabetes, cancer, leukemia, hypertension (high blood pressure) or hypercholesteremia (high cholesterol). In fact, it should be more of a global health concern than many of these diseases as obesity can lead to all of them. In other words, if you are obese you are more likely to develop: diabetes, cancer, hypertension, hypercholesteremia, a myocardial infarction (heart attack), a cerebral vascular accident (stroke), renal (kidney) failure, depression, etc. On the contrary, these diseases don't necessarily lead to obesity. What we do not know is that it is killing us. African-Americans must understand that obesity is the most extensive non-communicable disease in the African-American community. I often say, Obesity is doing to our community what hurricane Katrina did to New Orleans. We must therefore get rid of the number one health problem for African-Americans; obesity. Once we overcome obesity, we will then easily eliminate or gain better control of various other health problems that plague our community. The result? A life of peace, good health and longevity.

In order to do so, we must first change the way we think. We must be willing to undo what we have been doing for many years. Eating to live longer will take a great deal of sacrifice and commitment; just as it does to be a good lawyer, doctor, teacher, police officer, friend, husband, mother, Christian, Muslim, Jew, Hindu and Buddhist. Just as the Food and Drug Administration (FDA) and most religious groups have guidelines for eating, we must develop guidelines that are specific to our culture (as an African descendant now living in America) and genes. These guidelines must be appropriate for our environment and conducive to a healthy lifestyle.

I can't stress to you enough that we are literally *dying* as a result of how we are eating. We are making poor choices in selecting our foods, and it is having a long term detrimental effect on our health and well being. We must begin to treat our bodies as temples just as God has commanded, because "blessed are they that do His Commandments, that they may have the right to the tree of life, and may enter in through the gates into the city." (Revelations 22:14. Holy Bible, King James Version).

I have used scriptures from the Bible to provide us with spiritual support and guidance. It is my hope and prayer that this doesn't offend or alienate those of other religious backgrounds, as this is certainly not my intent. As a Christian and a physician, I often recall Jesus explaining to Satan that "man cannot live by bread alone but by every word that comes from the mouth of God." Proper eating and exercise must first be done under the direction of God and secondarily under the supervision of a God relenting and qualified professional (i.e. nutritionist, dietician or physician). For only God truly knows what is best for you. Whether you are Christian or not, it is innate for you to want a life filled with happiness and longevity. We all naturally want to be full of energy, free of disease as well as mentally and physically strong.

I believe that nature is proof that our Supreme Being expects nothing but the best for us. He has developed a system of perfection from which, man has unfortunately strayed. And as result of our disobedience, we have become a nation of extreme illness at the mental, physical, spiritual and emotional levels. As you read, I will introduce you to The Eat Right-Sunlight™ theory. This simple, yet essential premise describes the natural way of eating, and most importantly, the way our Ruler intends for us to eat. We must return to the laws of nature and natural living. The more natural we live, the more natural we become, and the closer we are to the original man and the way of life expected and commanded by God.

As a guide for the African-American community, I have also developed six steps to successful eating in order to live longer. Each step will be addressed individually and if adopted as a lifestyle, will enhance our knowledge base, advise us of our choices of foods and ensure a healthier and longer life.

SIX STEPS TO EATING TO LIVE LONGER

1. Learn Your Ideal Body Weight. Get There and Stay There.

2. Learn Your Family History.

3. Change Your Way of Thinking and Your Choice of Foods.

4. Change Your Level of Activity.

5. Educate Your Family and Friends on Proper Eating and the importance of Exercise.

6. Maintain This New Way of Living, Forever!

"The Lord said to Noah, Go into the boat with your whole family; I have found that you are the only one in the entire world who does what is right. Take with you seven pairs of each kind of clean animal, but only one pair of each kind of unclean animal". (Genesis 7:1-2, Good News Bible).

"Then the Lord said to Noah, "Go into the ark, with all your household, for you alone have I found righteous before Me in this generation. Of every clean animal you shall take seven pairs, males and their mates, and of every animal that is not clean, two, a male and its mate". (Bereshit (Genesis) 7:1-2, JPS Tanakh (Torah)).

The plan outlined in this book is not made only for you to read, but for you to study, discuss, live and triumph with. It is meant for you to begin a new walk up a path of discipline, cleanliness, greatness, excellence, success, spirituality and wholesomeness. The first step is to realize who you are, whose you are and that you are what you eat. Genetically, you are very similar to the original man, who was created by the originator and given the original diet. Our Torah and Bible teach us that certain foods were considered forbidden to eat (clean and unclean) before Noah, Abraham, Judaism, Christianity and Islam even existed. Just like Adam and Eve, you have been swindled into eating a food that will lead you down the path of unrighteousness, sickness and untimely death. With the completion of this book, I now have a tool to deliver this message of healthy living to my patients, churches, schools and the African-American community at large.

I can think of no better way to conclude this introduction than with a quote from Albert Schweitzer, a Nobel prize winning physician who was a pioneer in the study of the wellness of Africans (primitive man) and how their diet affected their well being. He was a missionary who quickly realized the importance of the genetically oldest human's diet and how this modern-day westernized cuisine is killing us:

> "On my arrival in Gabon (Africa) in 1913, I was astonished to encounter no cases of cancer. I saw none among the natives two hundred miles from the coast...I cannot, of course, say positively that there was no cancer at all, but, like other frontier doctors, I can only say that, if any cases existed, they must have been quite rare. This absence of cancer seemed to be due to the difference in nutrition of the natives compared to the Europeans..."

This concept of unclean food leading to disease has been around since the beginning of time and we seem to stay steadfast at not doing what's best for us. With our children becoming sick at an early age, with our adults living shorter and less independent lives, we must change. I therefore humbly present this book to those willing to accept my writings based on my research and experiences as a physician. This book is not intended to supersede the recommendations of your physician, make diagnoses or criticize the lifestyle of any particular group of persons. Although this book has referenced many biblical writings as it relates to health, I am a Christian that believes that no man should be judged by the food he eats, the drink he drinks or his way of worship (Colossians 2:16). I do, however, believe that we will be judged on, amongst other things, the respect we have for this shrine (of a body) that God has so graciously blessed us with. I am also a Christian who confesses that our bodies are temples of God and that we must put into them only the things that can be used for the uplifting and glorification of God. If any expression offends you or goes against the will of God, I ask in advance that I be forgiven by you and our Heavenly Father.

Chapter One

How It All Began: Evolutionobesity

"Beloved I wish above all things that thou mayest prosper and be in health, even as thou soul prospereth." (3 John 1:2. Holy Bible, King James Version).

If we took a snap shot of man shortly after God removed His hands of creation, what would we see? Where would we look? What would man's typical day consist of? What did we eat and drink? How long did we live? How did we die?

Evolutionobesity describes how we evolved from humans that could not store energy (fat), into those that could, and now are suffering from an excess of it.

It is no mystery to scientists that primary man developed on the land we now refer to as the continent of Africa. This advancement began several million years ago and we slowly evolved into modern day "me" and "you." During this process of fruition, we appreciated the untainted benefits of nature.

We lived in small groups and moved among the land in unity. Each member of the clan had a specific role. Before we became meat eaters, the entire family would collect fruits and vegetables that were found to be of great nutritious value. We drank plenty of water and enjoyed the wholesome juices from the tropical fruit we ate. When we became carnivores, the role of each tribe member changed. The men and boys spent their time in search of animal meat. Over the years, capture grew from primitive animal traps into fancy tools and weapons. Women and young girls became the exclusive gatherers.

Our bodies were free of cancers, hypertension, diabetes, obesity, degenerative arthritis, high cholesterol, and other modern day ailments. In addition to the righteous eating we did, we ran, swam, jumped, and played often. All of this was done while exposing our melanin rich skin to the sun to strengthen our body and make our challenging days easier to enjoy.

The term *evolutionobesity* is just as novel to you as it is to me. It is a term that I recently created in my quest to explain when and why man developed this heinous disease characterized by this excessive accumulation of fat, and all of its affiliated ailments such as diabetes, high cholesterol, heart attacks, strokes, arthritis, etc. The oldest human remains, according to a PBS publication entitled *Search for the First Human* (November, 2004), were found in Africa.[1] This group of ancestors called *Orrorin tugenensis* possessed full molars and small canines suggesting that the Orrorin often ate fruit and vegetables and only enjoyed animal flesh when available. Six million years ago, the body size of this early man was similar to that of a small chimpanzee. They had no fat accumulation, were moderately muscular and had smaller brains. Their facial bones were developed in such a way to accompany the attachment of thicker and stronger muscles for fast and aggressive chewing of their food. The availability of food however was few and far between.

In 1974, the remains of a prehistoric woman called "Lucy" were found in Africa as well. She lived some three million years ago and was part of a species called *Australopithecus*. She stood upright and walked on two feet (bipedal) just as we do today. Until the Orrorin remains were unearthed, she was considered to be our closest link to original man. While the Australopithecus are very closely linked to modern day man and bear much of the same physical and genetic make-up, they were much healthier than we are. At this stage, your descendants were not much different from the Orrorin although they lived about 3 million years after the Australopithecus. The primary foods were fruit, vegetables and animals, when obtainable.

Your ancestors evolved into a group of people not much different from you about 2 million years ago. The Homo Habilis were considered the first "true humans." They created and used tools they made from stones. They too lived in Africa and ate foods like the Orrorin and Lucy. It was during this time that your "people of the past" developed a taller body stature and their brains began to become larger and more developed. With the introduction of this new equipment, they were able to capture and kill animals more easily. In turn, they began to eat more animal flesh. Within 500,000 years of becoming the Homo Habilis, we began to make fire and use it for dietary advancements. This Homo erectus had mastered bi-pedalism and would now travel over large land bridges and across the waters in search of an even larger variety of foods. About one million years ago, this evolutionary state marked the spread of man across the entire world and the beginning of different races, cultures and ethnicities as we know them today. You were now considered true hunters and gathers as our brains evolved into a more complex and far more intelligent organ. Although it happened at a very slow pace, our development was only beginning.

As Homo sapiens and Neanderthals, you were now "wise men and women" that lived in African caves and huts ideally located near rivers and lakes. This allowed you to eat an abundance of fish, just as Jesus did. You developed fishing baskets and rods along with boats to better enjoy the gathering of your foods. You could also use your now even more advanced equipment such as spears, harpoons, scrapers, bow-and-arrows, cudgels and hand axes, to catch animals as they visited the waters to drink. Your community consisted of tribes of up to 100 people.

Fire was used more often to heat/cook foods and honey was used to sweeten foods. Unfortunately, Paleolithic man still went days to weeks without eating because food still was not always available. In order to have the energy to continue to fish, hunt, and gather, your body needed to develop a means of storing this food energy. This storage mechanism would be able to provide the body with the energy needed to continue to protect communities, build housing for growing populations (tribes, cities, states), climb trees to gather fruit, seize and prepare animal flesh, transport equipment while hunting and carry the gatherings back to their communities. The energy tank needed to be full enough to drive these developing bodies until an animal was hunted and the next fruit and vegetables were gathered.

Today, man has well evolved into an animal that has the ability to store energy as fat. This energy is measured in the form of calories. Fat is developed as a tissue known as adipose. Adipose tissue is made up of tiny fat cells called adipocytes. The number of fat cells one has is determined at birth and man's ability to increase the number of these fat cells exists for only a short period of time (until puberty). As an adult, man cannot produce additional adipocytes but can cause them to enlarge by consuming an excess of calories. This is how man has evolved into an animal that has the potential to become overweight or obese. As energy expenditure (i.e. running, walking) takes place, these cells shrink as does one's total body mass. Weight reduction therefore leads to a decrease in the size of the adipocytes but not the number of adipocytes.

At times when no food is available the process is reversed. The energy stored in these fat cells can be converted from the stored fat into glucose. Glucose is blood sugar and is the major energy source for our body. Fat is converted into glucose by an intracellular process our bodies developed called gluconeogenesis. Man's evolution into a fat storing creature also brought about an increased craving for meat and led to an even larger sized brain. This increase in brain size was directly related to the more complex human body that this brain now controlled. The brain in turn needed more "brain food" to function. This explains why we turned to a wider variety of food and began to travel outside of Africa to expand our menu. We began to search for plants that contained higher level of sugars and meats that were low in fat and high in protein. As our ability to reason further increased, so did our brain dimensions, height, hunting and gathering skills, reproductive ability, and food availability. This yielded a more refined civilization through natural selection and paved the way for modern man. We then began to breed cattle, trade with our ancestors that migrated out of Africa, draw, craft, carve, replace stone with copper bronze and iron, and become an agricultural society.

To better understand the influence of food and genetics on the evolution of obesity, one can look at modern day Asia, India and China know from first hand experiences what a chronic food shortage does to the body. After millions of deaths over the last fifty years, due to the lack of food, scientists were able to take a closer look at things. For thousands of years they were famished and undernourished. However, as their economies grew, so did their appetites. In the early 1970's, the Indian and Chinese population began to eat two to three times as much meat, sugar and fatty foods than ever before since early man inhabited that part of the world. Asians then transformed from an undernourished state to an over nourished state. With this change in diet and an increase in the rate of overweight and obesity, came a change in their body's ability to ward off disease such as cancers, hypertension and diabetes.

Chapter Two

Hunger

"I was hungry and you gave me food, I was thirsty and you gave me drink, I was a stranger and you welcomed me" (Mathew 25:30, Holy Bible, King James Version).

Hunger is a normal feeling that all animals experience when the body is in need of energy and essential nutrients (vitamins, minerals, fat, carbohydrates, protein, water, etc.). The feeling is often interpreted as an unpleasant feeling of distress that may even present as weakness. These feelings of survival-compromise start at a part of the brain called the *hypothalamus*. When you're hungry, the stomach muscles undergo intermittent painful spasms called hunger pangs. Man, the most advanced animal, can go up to 1-2 months without eating when our bodies are in good health. When Jesus was tempted by the devil, the biblical story tells us that he went forty days and forty nights without food.

Hunger seems to have an imposter that has a way of invading the thoughts and emotions of many of us. I refer to this false sense of craving for food as *false hunger*. Misinterpreting false hunger as true (or real) hunger is a major problem amongst African-Americans. Overweight, obese and female African-Americans seem to experience false hunger most often. The best way to distinguish between the two is to learn the differences and then be trained on how to recognize and resist false hunger. It has been a challenge for me to get patients to realize that often times their minds are crying out for emotional or financial support, rest, thirst quenching, love, excitement, companionship, affection, vacation time or respect but not food. Some patients have even tried to convince me that they are always hungry. These patients have been experiencing false hunger which is the desire for unnecessary or harmful foods in the absence of true hunger. If you are overweight or obese, you cannot afford to give in to false hunger any longer.

In my experience, the most common cause of responding to false hunger is emotional stress. When polled, many patients admit that their false hunger can be most commonly traced back to a form of stress. Food, in that sense, provides satisfaction and relieves the stress. Physiologically, this relief occurs through the actions of a chemical called serotonin. The second most common presentation of false hunger is out of habit. My patients eventually understand that when they routinely finish all of the food (regardless of their degree of hunger) served to them that they are often taking in an excessive amount of calories. I also help patients realize that when they eat a hefty "lunch" just because the clock struck noon, or eat ice-cream just because they just finished dinner, they may end up overweight or obese.

For overweight and obese people, hunger should be interpreted as a sign for you to provide only the amount of energy you will need to complete the work you will be doing for the next two to three hours. What do I mean? The average person burns approximately 150 calories per hour while sitting at a desk using a computer. If one does that between the hours of 9a.m. and noon, they may have burned only 450 calories (150 calories X 3 hours = 450 calories over 3 hours). Therefore, when they eat a meal at 8:00 a.m. it should be just enough calories to get through this task. That means, eating a morning/breakfast meal worth 800 energy calories is too much and the remainder will be stored as fat.

I once asked a patient of mine to spend 48 hours without looking at a watch or clock and without allowing his senses (seeing, hearing, smelling and touching) to be influenced by food. This patient, (we will call him Mr. Daniels), a 28 year old auto industry supervisor, was determined to get my point so he stayed in his home the entire following weekend. He watched no television and didn't listen to the radio (thereby eliminating all food commercials) and he prepared his own meals (smelled and touched no other foods). Because he used no time keeping devices, time couldn't dictate the onset of hunger or send false hunger signals. The following Monday he called me explaining that the first day was a challenge but the second day he ate food only because he knew he needed to eat something. Since then, Mr. Daniels has been able to recondition his thought process and he always asks himself, before he eats, if the food he is about to eat is for true hunger. For him, the best way to deal with these pseudo-hunger signals was to first experience it and then subjectively identify them. Incidentally, Mr. Daniel's body mass index (see Chapter 27 discussion on BMI) has decreased astonishingly from 41 to 24 within a twelve month period.

How To Recognize and Overcome
False Hunger:

1. _Understand the origin of your false hunger signals when they present themselves._ When you feel hunger, ask yourself if you just experienced a stressful event and assess your emotions for feelings of sadness or hopelessness. For example, are you hungry just because it's lunch time or are you craving popcorn just because you're watching a movie? A simple way to do this is to keep a 30 day log of how you feel and what you're doing whenever you feel hungry. Any patterns you notice are sure to be of false hunger origin.

2. _Never respond to hunger without first ruling out false hunger._ Putting food in your mouth shortly after deciding that you're hungry is a serious problem. Remember that Jesus sacrificed for over a month and proved that you've got plenty of time and

that these deceitful temptations can be overcome. Instead, try creating positive or rewarding thoughts or drink a glass or two of water (since you should be drinking one-half a gallon per day anyway). If your hunger persists, wait at least 30 minutes before reaching for something to eat. Over time, you will find that as the false hunger signals go away, so will your hunger because it was not real. You will literally forget about your cravings.

3. _Retrain your brain to not send the misleading signals_. After eating, if the food did not completely satisfy you, take away your hunger pangs or remove undesired emotions and weakness then it was probably not real hunger. Experiences of false hunger must never be forgotten. Record them on paper and in your mind's memory bank because they will be back. And when they do, this is when you must put on your full armor and fight it. Recognizing,

understanding and ignoring signals of false hunger will cause them to disappear and come less frequently. Your brain will no longer allow them to flourish. Like anything else, practice will lead to significant improvement and head toward perfection. Also, remember the food you eat must have nutritious value when assessing your hunger. For example, grab your favorite fruit instead of your favorite candy bar. The fruit will provide you with the nutrients your body desires with true hunger where junk foods don't, and the true hunger may therefore persist.

Meanwhile, try gauging true and false hunger by using my hunger scale. Use this while you sort things out between true and false hunger. The principle is simple: you rate your hunger on a scale from 10-100. 10 represents you feeling completely full and 100 represents you feeling very hungry.

10	20	30	40	50	60	70	80	90	100

False Hunger	True Hunger	High Risk & Trouble Zone

If you rate your hunger at 60, 70 or 80 then you are probably hungry enough to eat. You should always eat when your hunger is at this level. If you give your level of hunger a score of 90 or 100, you are too hungry and waited too long to eat. You are setting yourself up for weight gain when you flirt with this level of hunger. Eating at this level is very dangerous and you must pace yourself as it would be easy to overeat, gain weight and lose control. If you are at 50 or less on my hunger score index, then you aren't really hungry enough to eat. At this score, your hunger should always disappear after 20-30 minutes. It's time to become a hunger detective!

Another way I get my point across to my patients is by referring to a gas gauge. I ask my patients to consider their stomachs a gas tank except their stomach's tank should never be on empty or full. What I explain to them is that they should eat only when they are near the ¼ mark and only up to the ¾ mark. When dealing with true hunger, one should never wait until they reach the "E" level to eat. This will lead to binging. Conversely, you should never eat until you reach the "F" level as this will stretch the stomach. This will lead to eating more and lack of satisfaction.

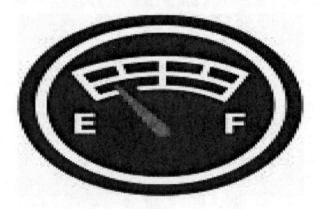

Eat and Live Longer Tip:

Only eat when your 'tank' is ¼ full, and always stop when you hit the ¾ mark!

Chapter Three

Soul Food

"What! Know ye not that your body is the temple of the Holy Ghost which is in you, which ye have of God, and you are not your own?" (1 Corinthians 6:19.Holy Bible, King James Version).

"Soul food had its purpose yesterday but today, has unfortunately become the deadly food of African-Americans," R. Eadie, MD.

When one becomes "Spiritual," "Saved," "Holy," a better person, more mature or develops a close relationship with their supreme being; one changes. Many of the things you did, you no longer have a desire to do. Your new way of life will be obvious by the new things you do. And, the way you walk, speak and carry yourself will tell your story. Your way of thinking changes by the divine intervention of God. Should not the way you eat also change? After all, Jesus' last meeting with the disciples was The Last Supper. The food you eat is obviously important.

The term *ethnic group* refers to a group or race of people that are classified according to their commonalities. Their culture can be understood by observing their race, religion, and social beliefs. When referencing African-Americans, one would first consider any American of African (and especially of black African) descent. A specific uniqueness about the African-American culture is that it is, at times, described as being one with "soul." That is, we are thought to have a strong and spiritual means of expressing ourselves through our music (e.g. Negro Spirituals), food, dance, hair styles, clothing, dialect, etc. "Soul food" is the ethnic food of African-Americans. Soul food has also been known as "slave's cuisine" and "good times" food. Nonetheless, this type of food has been part of the African-American culture since the early 1400's.

In order to properly define "soul food," one must first appreciate its history. Traditionally, African people would eat grains, legumes (pods, vegetables from the pea family), yams, sorghums, watermelons, pumpkins, okra, greens, eggplant, cucumbers, onions, garlic and a large amount of fruit. Meats would be served sparingly, as the average African ate a mostly vegetarian diet. When the slave trade began, it was also the start of a change in the diet of the African people, and the beginning of "soul food" as we know it today. Aboard the slave ships, the slave master would feed the slaves his left over food. The enslaved African became accustomed to eating a small serving of meat (soiled fishes), rice (covered with a slabber sauce), beans, and vegetables. Historically, this meal was their first exposure to a diet high in salt.

On the American plantation, the African was again forced to eat a "new plate." Their previously healthy African plate was quickly replaced with an unhealthy African-American dish. The slave's diet now consisted of the slave owner's throw away foods and the things he refused to eat. The vegetables were the tops of turnips, beets, and dandelions. Eventually, new types of greens (e.g. collards, mustards) were being cooked by the slaves. Now, the meat (pig's feet, ham hocks, chitterlings, pig's ears, hog jowl, tripe, and crackling,) became the main dish. If lucky, they would be given generous portions of greens and molasses (as dessert). The common drink suddenly became lemonade and iced tea.

The slave's diet deteriorated even more into this modern day "soul food" after we became the plantation house cooks. The skill and creativity of the slaves created plates covered with greasy fried chicken. In addition, sweet potatoes (in place of the African yams), and nuts were becoming the preferred taste. Dinner time, if granted by their master, was a time when the slaves would gather after a hard day of work. They would eat their "good times" foods, worship God and teach their youth about their wonderful life back in their motherland.

It was this "well appreciated" and "master-minded" soul food that gave rise to many popular dishes found today in restaurants across America. These popular dishes include hush puppies, gumbo, gut strut, croquettes, pot likker and many more. Soul food is even served in other ethnic restaurants in the form of appetizers and desserts. Soul food, as we know it today, is more than just a plate of creativity. To the

African-American, it is a symbol of tenacity, hardship, unity and blessings from God. Even now, it is eaten by African-Americans on a regular basis or during special gatherings (i.e. holidays, funerals, and parties).

Soul food is an outward sign of the inward grace of African-Americans. Soul food restaurants, to me, are businesses that exist only because of the selfishness of the slave master and the creativity of the slave. They are monuments that represent the birth of the African-American slave culture. Along with the creation of soul food came the beginning of many new diseases for the Africans transplanted in America. We began to see significant heart disease, cancers, strokes, diabetes and kidney disease. To the slave, eating soul food was a symbol of tenacity, hardship, unity, and a gift from God. But God has since then blessed our people and delivered us from slavery, yet we have not delivered ourselves from such awful eating. It served its purpose, but it was a bad food during a bad time. Today, on the other hand, to eat that type of food is an abomination and should be unheard of except in the history books relating to slavery and the advancement of African-Americans. We must strive for self preservation instead of self destruction. Again, we can do this by first changing the way we think. We have to want to live better, more prosperous and healthier lives. We must change what we eat and the way we eat. And that includes getting rid of or changing the contents of soul food.

Soul food is no different than drugs, alcohol, racism, poverty and unemployment in that it contributes to the destruction of African-Americans. Our bodies are God's temples and we must cook, eat, drink and serve foods that are righteous and godly. First Corinthians 3:16-17 says: "Know ye *not that ye are the temple of God, and that the spirit of God dwelleth in you? If any man defiles the temple of God, him shall God destroy; for the temple of God is holy....*" Since soul food is unhealthy and is responsible for much of our sickness and countless deaths, why then do we continue to eat it? Is it simply because it is a part of our culture or heritage?

I liken African-American people to Esau, brother of Jacob and son of Isaac. Africans are God's first born children and Esau was Isaac's first born son. The first born has access to the birthright. The birthright entitles one to the family inheritances, head of the household and many other blessings. As a people, we were given the most fertile land, precious treasures, wisdom, knowledge and bodies engineered to endure hardness like true soldiers. Esau was privileged to a double portion of his father's assets and would become the head of the family upon the death of his father. Esau one day returned home famished after he had been hunting in the wilderness. His brother Jacob had been cooking and Esau was tempted by the tantalizing aroma. Esau's desire for food proved to be his downfall as he traded his God-given blessings for food. Today, we continue to miss out on blessings as we eat food that is forbidden and that we know is destroying our bodies. We are preoccupied with satisfying our hunger instead of satisfying our bodies and our God. Several facts suggest that we have replaced worshiping God with the worship of food: many people get upset with me when I speak against soul food, most African-American adults are either overweight or obese, we adamantly refuse to give up beef or pork, fasting for 40 days seems impossible to us, we still eat what we eat even after being told that it is killing us, we don't eat the way Jesus ate.

The bottom line: The less you eat like your African ancestors, the more susceptible you are to disease, the faster you age, and the sooner you will die!

Chapter Four

The Geechee and The Gullah

"Ef oona dey frum de lowcountree an de islandt, lookya, e da time fa go bak. Disyah da wey fa cum togedda wid wi people fa hold on ta de tings wa wi peepol lef wi."

Our God-given, well-designed and nearly perfect way of life has been diluted and dismantled since our relocation to the United States and our adaptation of the "western way." Some of us have very little insight on our previous culture and how it relates to how we ate to live longer and had prosperous lives on our native soil. The state of South Carolina and Georgia still house a group of people who, because of their geographic isolation, have been able to preserve more of their African culture than any other group of African-Americans. These groups of people were referred to as Geechees and the culture (language, cooking style, arts, etc.) is referred to as Gullah. I doubt it very seriously if you can find any group of Americans more similar to ancestral Africans than the Geechees.

They came from western Africa (Sierra Leone, Liberia, Guinea, Guinea Bissau, Gambia and Senegal) to the "low country" of South Carolina and Georgia. Hilliard and Janie Eadie, my grandparents, were Geechee folk and they lived and died the Gullah way. In low country South Carolina, most of their African culinary skills were preserved along with the "foods of survival" they adopted during bondage. To the Geechee, rice, okra, grits, mullet, collard greens, sweet potatoes and boiled peanuts were African foods. Rice however, was their forte and having eaten it every day of my childhood, I can surely attest to that. In fact, South Carolina at one time produced most of this country's rice. An old school staple food for low country South Carolina was the Frogmore Stew with the Frogmore plantation on St. Helena Island (South Carolina) being its name sake. It consisted of the coastal crabs, sausage, potatoes, corn, shrimp (when available) and rice.

The Gullah dialect is considered a Creole language as it is a language that arose from contact between two or more different languages and consists of features of them all. According to *Gullah Pride*, it is specifically a mixture of Elizabethan English (16th and 17th century) and the following African tongues: Via, Mende, Twi, Ewe, Hausa, Yoruba, Ibo, and Kikongo.[1] Gullah was strategically spoken very rapidly. The faster they spoke the less the slave masters could understand. The Geechees that were isolated on islands in south east America maintained their African diets and way of life as best they could. Those who did this best lived much longer than those whose became more "Americanized."

My grandparents both died in their eighties. Although too early for my family, they lived longer than the average African American. Had they not eaten pork, fried foods, beef, dairy products and salty foods, they may still be here today. The result of them eating these types of foods was them suffering from hypertension, diabetes, cancer, congestive heart failure, high cholesterol and obesity. The Geechees that minimized this new way of eating lived to be much longer than my grandparents. *The State*, a Columbia South Carolina newspaper, published an article entitled *Saving Gullah*, where Sheila Middleton was quoted as saying; "I know people (Geechees) that are 95 and 100 who can tell me about my parents and grandparents."[2]

Mus tek cyear a de root fuh heal de tree.

Chapter Five

Butter, Margarine and Milk

"Of everything that goes inside of you, have a complete understanding of its effect on you."
R. Eadie, MD.

Many friends, family and patients have asked whether it is better to eat butter or margarine. This question is the reason why I have included this chapter in the book. They should instead ask me which one is *worse*. A clear and concise explanation must be provided to the masses so that they can understand my look of discomfiture and my delivery of a seemingly incomplete answer. Hopefully, the next few paragraphs will provide some "sunlight" on the situation.

Butter is made from animal's milk; today cow's milk is most commonly used. Today's cow is fed grains instead of grass and therefore has a newly altered fat content. Butter is doused with saturated fat (about 66% saturated and 34% unsaturated) and a lot of cholesterol. They both predispose you to atherosclerosis, inflammation, strokes, heart attacks, kidney disease and other untoward health problems. It also increases your omega-6 to omega-3 ratio (see chapter 9) which can cause the same problems.

Margarine, at one time, was made from beef fat, milk, chopped sheep's stomach and cow's udders. Today, it is made from vegetable and fish oils and is now used up to four times more than butter. Vegetable oils are mostly unsaturated and can therefore be marketed as being "heart smart." Unsaturated fats are liquid when refrigerated. So why is margarine a solid when it is in your refrigerator? Since the early 1900's, man has been converting these healthy oils (liquids) into solids. This means they have been converting these unsaturated (healthy) oils into saturated (unhealthy) oils through a process called hydrogenation. It is so called because hydrogen atoms are added to the oils. The other name for these bad fats is "trans-fats" as you will see them called on nutrition facts labels. While switching from butter to margarine may be a slightly healthier move, they both are similar in calories.

The truth of the matter is that both butter and margarine are bad for you. The answer to the question "which one is worse?" is *whichever one you use a lot of*. Yet, because of the elimination of saturated fats and its origin being from vegetables, margarine is the healthier choice between the two.

Now, on to Milk...The Merriam Webster's Medical Desk Dictionary defines Milk as a fluid secreted by the mammary glands of female animals for the nourishment of **their** young.[1] A more specific and modern day definition should be: an unwholesome liquid-meat usually extracted from a cow and intended for its young, but unnecessarily consumed by humans, rejected by the bodies of most Americans and implicated in promoting the onset of many human diseases, such as insulin-dependent diabetes mellitus, obesity, heart disease, cancers, strokes, Crohn's disease, asthma, ear infections, eczema and constipation.

There is only one thing that God can't do, and that is: make a mistake. He had a lot in mind when He created your beautiful dark skin, the big bright sun and foods enriched in calcium. How great Thou art! Your dark skin contains cells called melanocytes whose primary function is to produce melanin. Melanin is the dark pigment that is responsible for your skin color. The darker you are the more functional melanin you have. Sun rays interact with your skin and produce a premature form of Vitamin D. This chemical is transformed into active vitamin D by both your skin and your liver. This active vitamin D works as a hormone which increases the absorption of calcium in your intestines to build stronger bones. Naturally, the calcium comes from the food you eat.

Since 1940's, milk has been fortified (strengthened by the addition of) with vitamin D to reduce the incidence of rickets. Let me rephrase this, vitamin D is added to milk! Just as it is now added to orange juice, cough syrup, throat lozenges, etc. The truth of the matter is that exposure to sunlight for short regular intervals and proper eating is all we need to produce adequate vitamin D and calcium. God gave us natural ways of producing vitamin D while man gave us an unhealthy and ineffective way of obtaining vitamin D. The calcium in cow's milk is very difficult for us to use. This is especially true since it has a low magnesium level. Magnesium helps the body convert vitamin D, which the body needs in order to take advantage of bone strengthening calcium, into a form that it can use efficiently. By contributing to increased bone density, the mineral may help stall the onset of the debilitating, bone-thinning disease known as osteoporosis.

The Physicians Committee for Responsible Medicine writes: "It is a common myth that people should increase their calcium intake. Mostly, they are encouraged to take supplements and to drink more milk. But milk may not do a body good. The highest rates of osteoporosis are in the industrialized Western nations- the biggest consumers of milk."[2]

Generally, people think that drinking cow's milk is key to preventing osteoporosis, yet clinical research shows otherwise. The Harvard Nurses' Health Study trailed more than 75,000 women for over 10 years, and was unable to confirm a protective effect of milk consumption on broken bones.[3] Actually, increased intake of calcium from dairy products was associated with a higher incidence of broken bones. Another study done by a group of Australian researchers also showed that cow's milk increases bone fractures.

Moreover, African Bantu women eat a minimum amount of calcium per day. They also birth an average of nine children and breast feed them for up to two years. Yet, they never suffer from calcium deficiency and osteoporosis is almost nonexistent, even in women over 65 years of age.

All milk contains a sugar called lactose. This sugar is broken down by an enzyme called lactase. It shouldn't be hard to convince you that God intended for us to drink from our mother's breast until weaned. After being weaned off of milk, our bodies will naturally no longer produce lactase since we no longer need to drink any milk (from our mother's breast). Drinking another animal's (cow) milk makes most of us sick with a disease called lactose intolerance. In fact, being lactose intolerant is normal and being lactose tolerant is abnormal. Most of the world (over 75%) and up to 95% African-Americans cannot tolerate the lactose in cow's milk. If cow's milk was truly "nature's perfect food," then why does it sicken most of the world?

Lactose intolerance is at its highest frequency in some parts of Africa, East Asia, and among Native Americans but affects all mankind. It is now wrongly accepted that lactose intolerance is normal and lactose tolerance is abnormal or atypical. Northern Europeans usually have the lowest incidence of these dietary troubles. Given this distribution pattern of lactose intolerance, it is not surprising that dairy products are more popular among most Europeans but are rarely found in Asian and Native American households. What about the African-American households?

It is not healthy for us to drink another animal's milk. Human milk is for human babies, cow milk is for calves, and dog milk is for puppies. If the department of agriculture prepared a pig's milk with added vitamin D and spent billions of dollars promoting it as "a natural," placed it on a food pyramid, and told you to drink it, would you? Better yet, would you serve it to your children? Why is the human being the only adult animal that craves another animal's milk?

If child abuse is defined as the physical, emotion or sexual mistreatment of children, I submit to you that giving your child cow's milk could be a form of child abuse. Knowing that butter, cheese and milk are high in saturated fat, you are consciously predisposing your child to a higher risk of developing obesity, heart disease, diabetes, strokes, Mad Cow disease, multiple sclerosis, intestinal colic, intestinal bleeding, anemia, salmonella and many other bad diseases linked to milk drinking.

The process of pasteurization has turned out to be a problem. Pasteurization (heating cow's milk to kill bacteria) changes the natural quality of the proteins found in milk. This causes milk allergies in children and interferes with the ability to absorb the calcium inside of the milk. Homogenization of cow's milk is another process whose invention had good intentions but does the body NO GOOD. This process breaks the fat into very small particles that can easily be absorbed into the blood stream. This results in high triglycerides, cholesterol and clogged arteries.

Breast-feeding is the preferred method of infant feeding. Scientists are finally being honest with and advising that we give milk to our children with caution. Of recent, the American Academy of Pediatrics admitted that cow's milk should not be given to infants under one year of age. Instead, they should be breast fed. Medical research has demonstrated that breast-fed youngsters have higher intelligence, better social skills, stronger immune systems (thus fewer illnesses such as ear infections) and less allergies than their formula-fed peers. Dr. Benjamin Spock, author of the world-famous book *Baby and Child Care*, wrote in 1998, "Cow's milk is not recommended for a child when he is sick — or when he is well, for that matter. Dairy products may cause more mucus complications and cause more discomfort with upper respiratory infections."[4] This is of utmost importance for children with any respiratory disease such as asthma, bronchitis, bronchiolitis, pneumonia, etc. A major component to these diseases is the mucus plugging that occurs in the lungs.

Libraries, the internet and medical journals are filled with articles and other information opposing the intake of cow's milk by human beings. If you don't care to read them, simply listen to your body as it becomes sickened after you drink milk. Could it be because they know that the USDA and other government agencies allow a certain amount of contamination (pus, blood, antibiotics, pesticides, feces, etc.) to be present in the milk sold throughout our country. The crux of the matter is that God doesn't make mistakes. He made the breast so that it may produce milk. This milk is intended for the mother's newborn, not the newborn of a different mother or animal.

Finally, I have learned the detriments of milk from my personal experiences with it. As a child, I suffered from seasonal allergies, asthma, eczema, occasional hives, black rings around my eyes (shiners), red eyes, frequent bloating, gas and diarrhea. My doctor, mother and I had no idea that these symptoms were coming from my immune system's response to the proteins found in cow's milk. Some children may have reddish ear lobes or a glazed look in their eyes. Other symptoms that may be attributed to drinking the milk of a cow include bed wetting, lethargy, and inattentiveness. My body was rejecting this milk because I was allergic to it. Cow's milk is one of the most common food allergies experienced in childhood. There are many protein allergens in cow's milk that cause allergic reactions. Casein and whey are the two main components. Casein is a white, tasteless, odorless protein precipitated from milk by rennin. It is the basis of cheese and is also used to make plastics, glues and food. Casein accounts for over 80 percent of the protein in milk and is the most important allergen found in cheese. The harder the cheese, the more casein it contains. The curd that forms when milk is left to sour is called casein. The watery part which is left after the curd is removed is called whey. Whey accounts for the other 20 percent of milk protein.

Chapter Six

Free Radicals and Antioxidants

"...if thou wilt diligently hearken to the voice of the Lord thy God, and wilt do that which is right in his sight, and wilt give ear to his commandments, and keep all his statutes, I will put none of these diseases upon thee, which I have brought upon the Egyptians: for I am the Lord that healeth thee." Exodus 15:26. *(Holy Bible, King James Version).*

Oxidation is the process of adding oxygen to a substance. This reaction is always altering to the substance being oxidized. For example, metal oxidation produces rust while oxidation causes the banana to turn brown and then black. Oxidation causes green tea leaves to be converted to oolong or black tea leaves. And it is also why an apple turns brown after it is bitten or cut.

Within the human body, oxidation occurs with substances called free radicals. They can be helpful to man when they are produced by the body to help in digestion and the conversion of foods to energy (metabolism). In this

44

sense, they are helpful but they are generally very harmful since they are usually unstable molecules.

Free radicals are very unstable and highly reactive substances within your blood that have lost one electron and are aggressively looking for a replacement. They will attach themselves to any cell or molecule within your body to get the electron they lost. However, after combining to molecules that they shouldn't, they damage your cells or tissues. This can lead to cancer (DNA destruction), cardiovascular disease (blood vessel damage) and any other imaginable health problem, including accelerated aging (destruction of collagen causing your skin to sag). They are also produced when the body is exposed to harmful substances such as cigarette smoke, alcohol abuse, pesticides, cadmium, x-rays, gamma rays from radioactive material, car exhaust and industrial fumes. We are faced with over ten thousand free radicals per day. The good news is that many healthy foods provide substances called antioxidants that actually neutralize these free radicals, and render them harmless!

While your body already naturally produces antioxidants in order to help get rid of some of the free radicals present, it unfortunately does not produce enough to prevent disease. Therefore, we must make sure that we consume foods high in antioxidants. Major antioxidants that we can consume on a daily basis include vitamin A and beta-carotene, vitamin E, vitamin C and selenium.

- **Vitamin A and Beta-carotene:** Beta-carotene is a precursor to vitamin A. It protects green, yellow and orange fruit and vegetables from solar energy damage. Fortunately, it plays a similar role in the body. The carrots, squash, broccoli, sweet potatoes, tomatoes, kale, collards, cantaloupe, peaches and apricots that your grandmother insisted that you eat are rich sources of beta-carotene.
- **Vitamin E:** This vitamin can be stored with fat in the liver and other tissues. It delays aging, promotes healing of sunburns, etc. Natural food sources include

green leafy vegetables, vegetable oil and fish-liver oil, wheat germ, nuts, seeds and whole grains.

- **Vitamin C**: This powerful antioxidant cannot be stored by the body, so it is important to consume enough of it on a daily basis. This can be accomplished by eating the recommended amount of fruits and vegetables. Natural sources include citrus fruits, green leafy vegetables, strawberries, raw cabbage, green peppers, broccoli, and potatoes.
- **Selenium:** is a trace non-metallic element that resembles sulfur and tellurium and is used as a key component in photocopy machines. It is found in fish, meat and some cereals. It is a trace essential element that if low or absent can lead to many diseases. It is associated with a cardiomyopathy (disease of the heart muscle) in pregnant women, Coxsackie B infection, bowel disease, irregular heart rhythms, cardiac failure and cancer. Patients found to have low selenium levels often have a

Vitamin E deficiency as well. Following the foot prints of our ancestors, it is best to get selenium through foods, as large doses of the supplement form can be toxic. Healthy food sources include fish, shellfish, grains, eggs, chicken and garlic. Vegetables can also be a good source if grown in selenium-rich soils.

Chapter Seven

The Cow

"But the spirit saith expressly, that in later times some shall fall away from the faith, giving heed to seducing spirits and doctrines of demons, through the hypocrisy of men that speak lies, branded in their own conscience as with a hot iron; forbidding to marry, and commanding to abstain from meats, which God created to be received with thanksgiving by them that believe and know the truth. For every creature of God is good, and nothing is to be rejected, if it be received with thanksgiving: for it is sanctified through the word of God and prayer." 1 Timothy (4:1-5). (Holy Bible, Original African Heritage Edition).

This scripture doesn't mean that one is free to eat any type of animal meat. The above scripture specifies meats only which "God created to be received." This excludes meats that God created but did not expect us to receive (as food)! This scripture is often quoted or referred to when Christians defend their stance against vegetarianism or meat eating. The question that often surrounds this scripture is: what is the definition of meat? Meat is defined as the flesh of animals (including fish, birds and snails) used as food. In the Bible, the book of Luke (24:41-42) refers to fish as meat. In the book of Leviticus (11:2), we get directions on what animals men should eat and what animals men are advised to stay away from. Leviticus (7:23-27) also warns us against eating fatty foods. Since a Christian should live his life as Jesus Christ did, other questions often asked include: Did Jesus eat beef? And, what would Jesus eat? I don't think it is simply a coincidence that Jesus began his mission by gathering men (His disciples) that specialized in the catching of fish. He could have started with cattlemen, herdsmen, shepherds or some other occupation related to animals. The first four men called to accompany Jesus were fisherman. That leads me to believe that fish was a commonly eaten food and that it was more than likely the food of choice for Christ.

Although the Bible doesn't specify Jesus' diet per se, the aforementioned verse in the book of Luke (24:42) states that Jesus ate fish. In the book entitled *What Would Jesus Eat?*, Don Colbert suggests that beef was not a part of Jesus' diet.[1] The book explains how the American beef industry has a 200 year legacy. Beef is second to chicken when it comes to the American's choice of meat. It has played an integral part in the nation's growth, economic prosperity and failing health. According to a survey done by the USDA Economic Research Service in 2005, the average American eats about 67 pounds of beef per year. African-Americans, arguably the unhealthiest group of Americans, eat about 77 pounds of beef per person per year. Hispanics were found to eat an average of 69 pounds of beef per year; whereas Caucasians eat 67 pounds and 62 pounds are eaten by other races.[2] They also found that low-income Americans also tend to eat more beef than consumers in higher income households. Does that suggest that beef is for the poor and leads to poor health? Dr. James Howenstine, author of *"A Physicians Guide to Natural Health*

Products that work," had the following answer to this question:

"Discontinuing or decreasing the intake of meat - particularly beef - appears to be a sensible health measure as it could improve immune function leading to more effective resolution of infections and killing of cancer cells. Current concepts about cancer believe that all persons are identifying and killing multitudes of cancer cells as long as their immune system is healthy. Removing the detrimental immunosuppression caused by excessive iron deposition in the body seems likely to improve the performance of our immune systems. Persons not wishing to give up eating meat can probably stay out of trouble by donating blood regularly, which should remove the excess dietary iron. Decreasing the intake of meat - particularly beef - may decrease the risk of both heart attack and cancer."[3]

The cow has always played a role in human life in one way or another. In Africa, the cow's primary function was to serve as a draught animal (pulling plows, carts, etc.). Not many cows were raised in Africa because of its very warm climate and scarcity of grasslands. If Africans did eat the flesh of the cow, it was done very sparingly. In America, the cattle industry developed in the 1800's after Joseph "the real" McCoy became a livestock trader. He transported longhorn cattle from Texas to Chicago and then to the eastern boarders. Some consider them the oldest form of wealth in the United States. Their ability to provide meat and dairy while reproducing themselves and eating nothing but grass has furthered human interest to raise and sell them. They are called ruminants, meaning they have a unique digestive system that allows them to synthesize amino acids. This allows them to survive on grass and other vegetation. The cow is a low maintenance source of food and income.

Today, beef should not be offered a spot in the kitchen or on the plates of African-Americans. Beef is very high in fat, full of damaging chemicals and is destroying America's "black" race. The type of fat that is present in beef is mostly saturated fat. It is the saturated fat that clogs the arteries of African-

Americans and contributes to heart attacks, strokes and kidney failure. Beef fat becomes saturated because the bacteria in the ruminant stomach of the cow hydrogenates, or saturates, the fats within the plants that cows eat. Could this be why the leading cause of death among Africa Americans is heart disease? Also, packaged beef from your local grocery store has an added ingredient called sodium nitrite which is a known cancer causing agent. Could this be why cancer is our second leading cause of death?

As if that isn't convincing enough, recent news reports remind us of the beef eater's risk of getting infected with the infectious protein that causes mad cow disease. Furthermore, beef is often obtained from cow's that are fed chicken litter, animal parts, crops sprayed with pesticides and other highly toxic substances that don't belong in the body of a cow or man.

It also appears that God doesn't want us to eat the flesh of meat eating animals. Animals that eat meat are considered scavengers. Scavengers will eat anything, especially the dead animals they find on the ground or at the bottom of waters. Their other purpose is to clean up waste products of animals just like the algae eater in your home fish tank. The scavenger has the ability to introduce diseases that destroy some, if not all, of the organs in our bodies. As a reminder, the pig, catfish, carrion vulture, crabs, clams, oysters and lobsters are some the scavengers that the Bible forbids us to eat. The cow is "normally" a vegetarian animal and approved for human consumption; however, has now become a meat eating animal. After cow's are slaughtered, the remains of the cow are used in the production of cattle feed. Hence, they are meant to be herbivores but are transformed into carnivores. This is how cattle get mad cow disease. Man, after eating this infected cow, is at risk for acquiring the human form of mad cow disease called Creutzfeldt-Jakob disease.

The Prion

"My wounds stink and are corrupt because of my foolishness. I am troubled; I am bowed down greatly; I go mourning all the day long. For my loins are filled with a loathsome disease: and there is no soundness

in my flesh." (Psalm 38:5-6. Holy Bible, King James Version).

A prion is an infectious microscopic protein particle, similar to a virus, thought to be responsible for certain diseases that affect the nervous system. Many of us have never heard of a prion, but have heard of the diseases that it allegedly causes: Bovine Spongiform Encephalopathy or Mad Cow Disease, CJD (Creutzfeldt-Jakob Disease), Scrapie and Kuru. I often think of the prion as being immortal since it is essentially impossible to kill. Even with extreme heat, this tenacious protein survives.

Bovine Spongiform encephalopathy, another name for mad cow disease, was named in a simple and straight forward manner. The word bovine means cow. The spongiform was added to describe the sponge-like hole found in the brains of these sick cows. Encephalopathy plainly refers to the bizarre behavior that the cow displays once infected by the prion. The name mad cow disease is an even simpler name as it too gives reference to the cow's crazy behavior before it dies. Mad cow disease is a fatal disease which usually wipes out the cow within weeks. Along with the sponge-like pattern within the infected cow's brain, scientists have also described a pattern of nerve degeneration.

Since the prion doesn't live on plants, and cows are vegetarians, how do they get exposed to one another? The answer is frightening but true. As I mentioned previously, the cow is fed the body parts of other cattle and sheep (e.g. the brains, bones, muscle, blood, etc.). After being slaughtered, the remains of cows and sheep are turned into sausage and also added to the feed of other animals. The cattle eat their feed and get exposed to the prion (if present). It takes up to 7 years for the cattle to show symptoms of mad cow disease. You probably recall this disease running rampant through Europe in the 1980s and 1990s. Even worse, in December 2003 the U.S. secretary of agriculture announced that mad cow disease had been found in America.

Some 3600 years ago, God gave man Law on what we should and should not eat. One of the things mentioned in your Bible is to not eat the meat of scavenger animals and Mad Cow Disease is another reason why. The cow, because of the way man feeds it, is a scavenger. Scavengers are specially designed by God to be able to eat dead and decaying things. They help to keep the earth clean and free of diseased and dying animals. Some of them also eat the waste products of other animals. When we eat animals that are scavengers we take into our bodies all the infected food they have eaten. As you know, our bodies are not designed to handle this type of food. God, the most intelligent, gave us these laws because He loved us and wanted us to live long and healthy lives. Lives that are free of ailments such as Mad Cow disease. The obedient will never have to worry about this or many other diseases. I have been advising our community for almost a decade yet no one seems to want to hear about God's law as it relates to the foods we choose to eat.

In the early 1920s, H.G. Creutzfeldt and A. Jakob first described it as a rare and fatal neurodegenerative disease of unknown origin. It was later seen in people that inhabited the mountains of New Guinea. They practiced cannibalism and were thought to be infected after eating infected human flesh. This disease was called Kuru. Since this tribe doesn't exist anymore, neither does Kuru. Today, Creutzfeldt-Jakob disease (CJD) is what you have to worry about if you are a meat eater. The prion has been found in sheep, goats, mink, cows, mule deer and cats. If you eat an animal infected with the prion, you get CJD. So far, Creutzfeldt-Jakob is rare but is invariably fatal. There is no single test to diagnose it and no cure for the disease. Even cooking your beef well done doesn't destroy the prion. Ninety percent of those infected will die within 1 year.

Scrapie is the name of the disease designated to the sheep once it is exposed to the prion. Scrapie was first described in 1730 after observing sheep scraping themselves against objects. They would subsequently walk with a staggered gait, stop eating and die.

KRS-One, of Boogie Down Productions, shared his thoughts on eating beef and how it negatively affects members of our community in his 1990 hit, *"Beef"*:

"Let us begin now with the cow
The way it gets to your plate and how
The cow doesn't grow fast enough for man
So through his greed he makes a faster
plan
He has drugs to make the cow grow
quicker
Through the stress the cow gets sicker
Twenty-one different drugs are pumped
Into the cow in one big lump
So just before it dies, it cries
In the slaughterhouse full of germs and
flies
Off with the head, they pack it, drain it,
and cart it
And there it is, in your local supermarket
Red and bloody, a corpse, neatly packed
And you wonder about heart attacks? "[4]

If you have not heard or read the lyrics to this song in their entirety, I suggest that you take a look (or listen)...you cannot help but be enlightened and make better decisions about your food choices once you know the truth!

Chapter Eight

Fatty Foods

"The Lord gave Moses the following regulations for the people of Israel. No fat of cattle, sheep, or goats shall be eaten. The fat of an animal that has died a natural death or has been killed by a wild animal must not be eaten, but it may be used for any other purpose." (Leviticus (7:22-24). Good News Bible. Good News Translation)

Talking about fat, particularly body fat, with many of my male friends has always been a challenge. Often times I would be accused of "losing my blackness" when I would suggest that our women's large hips, buttocks and breasts could be a sign of unhealthiness. Excess fat is excess fat, no matter how you look at it. With time, these same women become overweight and then obese and eventually begin to hate their bodies. This "thickness" leads to diabetes, high cholesterol, heart attacks, strokes, cancer and kidney failure. These fat deposits come from an unhealthy diet. It is important to know the different types of fats... which fats are good, and which fats are bad. Foods high in fat produce bodies high in fat. The Greeks called fat *lipos*, hence the word lipids which we use to refer to this family of chemicals. Lipids, in the liquid form, are referred to as oils whereas lipids in the solid form are referred to a fat.

The fats found in foods are simply a combination of fatty acids. These fats are categorized as: saturated fat, unsaturated (mono and poly) fats and trans-fat. A saturated fat is a solid at room temperature and gets harder when chilled. It is called "saturated" because it has a hydrogen atom at every available carbon link in its chain. Butter, margarine, and fats in meat (e.g. beef) and dairy products are all especially high in saturated fat. Unsaturated fats are liquid at room temperature and get thicker when chilled. They are called "unsaturated" because they don't have hydrogen atoms at every available carbon link in its chain. If it drops one hydrogen atom it is called a monounsaturated fat. If it drops more than one hydrogen atom it is called a polyunsaturated. The more hydrogen atoms present, the more saturated the fat. The more saturated the fat, the more unhealthy the fat. Hence, monounsaturated and polyunsaturated fats do not raise blood cholesterol levels. Flaxseed oil, canola and olive oil contain the highest proportion of monounsaturated fat compared with other cooking oils.

To preserve the shelf life of certain foods, man has developed the process of hydrogenation. Hydrogenation is the process of adding hydrogen to unsaturated fats to make them saturated. Doing so raises your cholesterol, promotes obesity and causes cancers. It also lead to clogged arteries, strokes, heart attacks and promotes further illness by increasing bad cholesterol (LDL) and decreasing good cholesterol (HDL). Margarine is an unsaturated fat so one would expect for it to be a liquid at room temperature. However, it has undergone hydrogenation and was therefore converted into a saturated fat.

As of January 1, 2006, the Food and Drug Administration mandated that Nutritional Facts labels list the amount of trans-fats is in each food product. Anything more than 0% promotes death. Just as you decipher the newspaper, your monthly bills and your favorite novel, you must translate the Nutrition Facts Label on your foods into life or death (see chapter 31).

Cholesterol is a waxy-like greasy substance that provides absolutely no calories, therefore no energy. It is derived from the foods you eat and it is a very import substance in the body as it is a precursor to vitamin D and steroid hormones, protects cell membranes, enables you to absorb vitamins (E, A, D, K) and is needed for nerve cell communication. Your total cholesterol level is equal to your: LDL + HDL + Triglycerides. As a general rule, an adult's total cholesterol should be less than 200 mg/dl. Make sure your doctor has you take a cholesterol screening test on your next visit. Your doctor should order a lipid profile which includes:

- **LDL** (low density lipoprotein cholesterol, also called "bad" cholesterol). It is called bad cholesterol because it takes fat into the walls of your arteries which can lead to a clot formation, blockage and inflammation. This level should never exceed 130 mg/dl. **The lower the better**.
- **HDL** (high density lipoprotein cholesterol, also called "good" cholesterol). It is called good cholesterol because it takes the fat out of the blood vessels and into to the liver where it can be processed and eliminated. This level should always exceed 40 mg/dl. **The higher the better**.
- **Triglycerides** are fats carried in the blood from the food we eat. Excess calories, alcohol or sugar in the body are converted into triglycerides and stored in fat cells throughout the body. This level should never exceed 160 mg/dl.

In general, when your HDL is high and your LDL is low, you have a healthier heart and body. When the converse is present, your doctor should prescribe a change in activity, diet and sometimes medications. Ways to increase your HDL include, but are not limited to:

- Increase your exercise
- Decrease your animal fat intake (beef, lamb, veal, pork and whole-milk and dairy products)
- Decrease foods that contain tropical oils (palm, kernel, coconut)
- Eat less eggs and shrimp
- Eliminate saturated fats from your diet as much as possible
- Increase your soluble fiber intake (vegetables, fruit)
- Maintain a normal Body Mass Index (BMI)
- No cigarette smoking

The fact that the leading cause of death in America is coronary heart disease is not a novelty. But, America's understanding of how fatty foods contribute to our health is a new concept that must not be ignored in order to prolong our lives. It must be understood, accepted, and then cultured by all American families to combat childhood obesity as well. What we eat should promote life and longevity, not death. Let's stop the cycle of ignoring our increasing rate of heart attacks, strokes, cancers, kidney failure, diabetes and other diet related diseases. Let's make the decision to live!

Chapter Nine

Oils and the Powers of Fish

"Throw your net out on the right side of the boat, and you will catch some." So they threw the net out and could not pull it back in, because they had caught so many fish. *(John 21:6.* Good News Bible, Good News Translation).

The power of fish oils have been known since man has been eating animals. Different types of animals were eaten for different reasons. Even the Bible reminds us of this in 1 Corinthians (15:39): "All flesh is not the same flesh, but there is one kind of flesh of men, another flesh of beasts, another of fish, and another of birds." And, even after Jesus was crucified, buried & had risen, He reminded his disciples of what they should be eating. When His spirit no longer needed food for nutritious support, He asked for food. "He said this and showed them His hands and feet. They still could not believe, they were so full of joy and wonder; so He asked them, "Do you have anything here to eat?" They gave Him a piece of cooked fish, which He took and ate in their presence (Luke 24:40-43. Good News Bible, Good News Translation). He could've asked for cow, goat or chicken. He was obedient to Jewish dietary laws and would never to ask for pig flesh. Instead, He asked for fish. What He was interested in was the healthy benefits of eating fish. Did He want us to know the benefits of the omega-3 fatty acid?

The initial apostles were fishermen. He began his recruiting on the shores of Galilee where He was probably fishing as well. Could this be why the fish is the symbol of Christianity? Remember, the word ichthus comes from **Iota Chi Theta Upsilon Sigma** which is Greek for fish. That is an acrostic (a series of lines or verses in which the first, last, or other particular letters when taken in order spell out a word, phrase, etc.) which has the translation (in English) of *Jesus Christ, Son of God and Savior*. The fish symbol was also a way to secretly identify Christians during times of their persecution.

Let's take a look at what He may have wanted us to know about the benefits of the fish:

Omega-6 and Omega-3 are two types of fat. They are classified as polyunsaturated fatty acids to be more specific. Millions of years ago our diet provided us with a balanced amount of Omega-6 and Omega-3. In other words, the ratio of Omega-6 to Omega-3 was 1:1 or 2:1. This balance is what kept man from developing certain cancers, pains and inflammation at our joints & muscles, heart attacks and extreme fatigue, to name a few. This anti-inflammatory, anti-cancer & heart protecting combination no longer exist. The so-called agricultural and industrial revolutions have changed these ratios. Today, the typical American has increased this ratio because of the high levels of Omega-6 we consume. The modern day ratio went from 1-2:1 to 25-50:1. This ratio means increased damage to the cells, tissue and organs in your body.

Our new westernized diet has had profound effects on our families, friends, health and our community as a whole. Our Godly way of eating has been ignored. Like Adam and Eve, we continue to eat the forbidden. Not only that, we have altered, reconfigured and mutated the foods that were approved for eating (i.e. the cow). The consequence of such Godlessness is the same as other sinful acts; death.

Omega-6 (linolenic acid) and Omega-3 (alpha-linolenic acid) are essential fatty acids (EFAs), meaning their consumption is absolutely necessary for survival. They have been found to control the genes that regulate our metabolism. In plain English, they regulate the amount of fat you have in your body. This is done by reversing insulin resistance (stops diabetes), preventing fat storage (halts additional weight gain) and increasing the breakdown of fat (weight loss). As partners, they also lower your blood fat and cholesterol level, reduce all inflammatory reactions, lower blood pressures, prevent blood clotting, stop formation of cancerous cells and decrease your risk of heart disease.

On the other hand, if they are not partnered (1:1) and one out numbers the other, the reverse actions will occur. You will be more prone to weight gain, having high blood levels of cholesterol and other fats, becoming diabetic, having easily clotting blood, cancer, suffering from high blood pressure and heart attacks.

Today, because of the way we eat, we have an excess of Omega-6. Our problem is that we lack Omega-3. For example, pecans have about 21 grams of Omega-6 for every 1 (21:1) gram of Omega-3. Cashews have a 47.6:1 ratio; sunflower seeds have a 472.9:1 ratio where almonds have no omega-3 at all. Again, most of our diet has a ratio of at least 20:1 and this is proving to be deadly.

Thousands of years ago, because we ate high levels of green plants, fruits, nuts, berries, fish and lean meat, non-processed cereals (wheat, corn and rice) and refined oils, we lived healthier lives. The wild animals we ate had high levels of Omega-3. The animals we eat today have low levels of Omega-3 and high levels of Omega-6 because they are fed with grains (high Omega-6/low Omega-3). Current recommendations seem to suggest that we replace healthy oils with oils filled with saturated fat. Again increasing our Omega-6 levels while lowering our Omega-3 levels. Cottonseed oil has a ratio of 258:1, grape seed oil is 696:1, corn oil is 83:1 and peanut oil has no Omega-3.

Nutritional advice to eat a low-fat high carbohydrate diet, as you now see, can be misleading. The goal, instead, should be for us to consume fats that are high in Omega-3 and low in Omega-6 and saturated fats. Also, we must increase our intake of Omega-3 by consuming more fish (e.g. mackerel, herring, sardines, trout and salmon) just as Jesus did. Please keep the high mercury levels in mind, as many ocean fish are known to contain certain levels of mercury that can be dangerous, even fatal, if consumed in excess. If this is not plausible, then we MUST take daily molecularly distilled or purified Omega-3 supplements to balance the large amount of Omega-6 we now consume on a daily basis. The active fatty acids found in Omega-3 (fish oil) supplements are eicosapentaenoic acid (EPA) and docosahexaenoic acid (DHA). We should consider taking 2 grams of EPA and 1 gram of DHA supplements every day, so that we will live the healthy life that our God intended.

Omega-6 to Omega-3 Fat Ratio in Nuts & Seeds

Nuts and Seeds are highly recommended food items in your daily pursuit of eating to live longer. Remember that although nuts and seeds contain "good" fats, they are still high caloric fat! So, if you also have a goal of losing weight while eating right, you should limit your intake of nuts and seeds to no more than 2 servings per day. Below is a chart listing types of nuts and seeds and their ratio of Omega-6 to Omega-3. Use this information when deciding which to purchase for you and your family. Remember, the lower the Omega-6 to Omega-3 ratio, the healthier the nut or seed.

Nut or Seed	Omega-6 to Omega-3 Ratio
Walnut	4.2
Macadamia nuts	6.3
Pecans	20.9
Pine nuts	31.6
Cashews	47.6
Pistachio nuts	51.9
Hazel nuts (filberts)	90.0
Pumpkin seeds	114.4
Brazil nuts	377.9
Sunflower seeds & Almonds	Extremely high; no omega-3
Peanuts (a bean)	Extremely high; no omega-3
Pumpkin seeds	114.4

Chapter Ten

Soft Drinks

"Someone will say, "I am allowed to do anything." Yes; but not everything is good for you. I could say that I am allowed to do anything, but I am not going to let anything make me its slave." (I Corinthians 6:12. Good News Bible, Good News Translation).

Soft drinks, also called soda and pop, have been around for hundreds of years. They originated from soda water which has actually been around since the late 1700s. Soda was considered healthy and was simply a combination of water, lemon and honey. This was all natural and not bad as a beverage choice. The first cola-flavored beverage was introduced in the late 1900s. With African-Americans being major soda pop consumers, we must know the contents of what we're drinking. In the early 1900s, cola drinkers were unaware that it contained extracts of cocaine as well as caffeine-rich kola nut; hence the name COKE. Coke is also the street name for cocaine. Incidentally, I often refer to soda pops as liquid crack.

Which one does more harm to the African-American community overall? Today, most African-Americans don't know the ingredients of the soda pop they consume on a daily basis nor do we know what this "refreshing" drink does to our bodies.

Caffeine, like sugar, morphine, ecstasy, tobacco and nicotine, is a drug and has detrimental effects on your body. According to a John Hopkins Medical Center publication entitled *Caffeine and Health*, caffeine use is associated with several distinct psychiatric syndromes: caffeine intoxication, caffeine withdrawal, caffeine dependence, caffeine-induced sleep disorder and caffeine-induced anxiety disorder.[1] Individuals with various conditions such as generalized anxiety disorder, panic disorder, primary insomnia and gastro-esophageal reflux disease should never drink soft drinks. Those that are pregnant or suffer from urinary incontinence should be advised to reduce or eliminate regular caffeine use. As far as your heart is concerned, caffeine produces an increase in blood pressure and studies have established that caffeinated and decaffeinated coffee contains lipids, which raises your total cholesterol.

Just like with cocaine and alcohol, your body can become dependent (the state of relying on or needing it to function) on caffeine. A decrease or the lack of caffeine, like cocaine and alcohol, can therefore lead to withdrawal. Caffeine withdrawal affects both children and adults. Commonly reported symptoms include, but are not limited to: headache, fatigue, sleepiness, drowsiness, poor concentration and transient learning impairment. For children, this becomes particularly important as it relates to school. Your child may have a slow start in the morning and experience difficulty in staying attentive and comprehending because of the caffeinated soda you allow him or her to drink.

According to the Center for Science in the Public Interest, carbonated soft drinks are the single biggest source of calories in the American diet, providing about 7 percent of calories; adding in noncarbonated drinks brings the figure to 9 percent.[2] Teenagers get 13 percent of their calories from carbonated and noncarbonated soft drinks. Because of the sugar content in soft drinks, it is often referred to as liquid candy. A regular 12 ounce can of Mountain Dew, for example, has 46 grams of sugar. That is equal to 11 teaspoons of sugar in one single can. I highly recommend that you pour 11 teaspoons of sugar on your kitchen table and make it a topic of discussion for you and your family over dinner. You all should then decide whether or not you think this is a reasonable amount of sugar for you or your family to drink, ever! While you are looking at your table with this unhealthy pile of sugar on it, ask yourself: how much weight is that amount of sugar equivalent to if you drink one can of soda on a daily basis for one year? Eleven teaspoons of sugar is equal to 184 calories. And, there are 3500 calories in a pound. Therefore, one can of regular Mountain Dew per day for a year is equivalent to 20 pounds. Isn't that an unhealthy enough reason to not purchase it?

Just as you watch your children closely for any peculiar behaviors suggesting illicit drug usage, so should you for the drinks they consume. And please watch very closely. The empty calories consumed by us and our children contribute to many of our health problems, especially diabetes, overweight and obesity. Let's take a look at Diabetes, or "sugar" as it is commonly called within the African-American community. One type of Diabetes was once called childhood diabetes because its onset occurred at a young age. The other type of diabetes was called adult diabetes because it usually occurred during middle age. The adult onset diabetes is now called type 2 diabetes because it is now occurring at an alarming rate during childhood. Therefore, the childhood onset diabetes is now called type 1 and the adult onset type 2. There is an abundance of literature and scientific evidence to support the fact that soda pop leads to the onset of diabetes as well as overweight, obesity, osteoporosis, kidney stones, attention deficit hyperactivity disorder, tooth decay and other health problems. A major problem, however, is that the Food and Drug Administration doesn't require soft drink producers to list such warnings on their labels. The soft drink industry spends hundreds of millions of dollars yearly to get you, your friends and your family to become addicted to their product without considering the untoward health penalties.

The fizz and bubbles that you see and hear when you open your bottle or can of pop is the escape of pressurized carbon dioxide. As human beings, our bodies normally use oxygen for energy production and its metabolic waste product is carbon dioxide. An excessive amount of carbon dioxide, in the blood of a human, causes a metabolic disorder, increased sickness and eventually death. You got it, a substance that *when in excess kills us*, is added to the liquids that many of us have come to crave on a daily basis. The fact that we drink the very chemical that our bodies try very hard to eliminate was enough to keep me away from soda pops.

An appropriate definition for the word diet should be: *a nutritional act or food item designed to improve a person's physical condition or to prevent or treat disease.* Based on this definition of diet, diet soda pops are not true diet drinks! When my patients ask me if diet soft drinks are acceptable, my answer is usually YES and NO. I say yes not because I feel that diet pop is a good choice, but because I realize that I am being asked that question by someone who has probably been addicted to pop for a long time.

For those trying to lose weight, diet pop is a much better choice. My patients would be more successful at losing weight by eliminating the hundreds of unnecessary calories found in pop while they transition into healthy eating habits and behaviors. Realizing that knowledge is power, I slowly advise that they research and learn the effects that artificial sweeteners and diet sodas have on the human body. They are usually quick to remind me that diet soft drinks are usually low in sodium and is no significant source of fat (saturated, unsaturated and trans) calories. I then remind them that diet sodas are also not a significant source of fiber, vitamins, calcium, protein or iron. And, that they are carbonated drinks, likely to contain artificial food colorings, aspartame (see chapter 17 on artificial sweeteners), phosphoric acid, citric acid and caffeine in it as well.

Physicians, patients, mothers, fathers, aunts, uncles, sons, daughters, and friends alike must speak out against these detriments. We must ensure that our schools are not laced with vending machines that allow our children access to soft drinks. Organizations must not be allowed to sell or serve our children soft drinks. We must also educate our loved ones and community members of the harm that these new (foreign and not a part of our original diet) drinks are causing. Finally, we should encourage state and local governments to impose taxes on soft drinks and use the funds towards educating our children on how to eat and live longer.

Chapter Eleven

The Empty Calories of Alcohol

"But now I have written unto you not to keep company, if any man that is called a brother be a fornicator, or covetous, or an idolater, or a railer, or a drunkard, or an extortioner; with such a one know not to eat." (1 Corinthians 5:11. Holy Bible, King James Version)

For many years, I believed that the "beer belly" of my beer drinking friends began to develop as a direct result of the excessive amount of beer they drank. But, after spending several years working in inner-city Emergency Departments, I noticed that most alcohol users didn't have such oversized abdomens. And, since most "heavy" drinkers often deprive themselves of food during binges, it had to be more than the alcohol that caused this abdominal obesity. I then took a closer look at alcohol metabolism and focused on the byproduct acetate. Alcohol is first broken down to acetaldehyde. Acetaldehyde is a toxic substance and is thought to be responsible for the symptoms of hangovers. Acetaldehyde is further broken down into acetate.

Acetate is a substance that can be used by the body for energy in lieu of glucose. In the presence of acetate, the body will use it as its energy source instead of converting fat into glucose. So, eating any food during or near the consumption of alcohol will result in the storage of the food glucose (as fat). Again, this happens because the body is using the acetate from the alcohol as its fuel instead of the usual glucose. The body burns 73% less fat after consuming alcohol. This is certainly not to suggest that you should stop eating food while drinking alcohol. Instead, one should stop drinking alcohol.

Alcohol, like table sugar, is a well known naked food. It gives you sugar energy, but no nutrients. Alcohol (beer, wine and spirits) contains 7 calories for each gram consumed. Carbohydrates and proteins contain only 4 calories per gram while fat contains 9 calories per gram. Therefore from a caloric standpoint, alcohol consumption is very similar to fat consumption. Yet, after it is converted to acetate and used as energy, only about 5% of the alcohol calories are converted into fat. Every food substance you eat provides calories, thus some form of energy. But, not all calories come with the amino acids, fatty acids, vitamins, minerals and fiber our bodies need. Such foods are also called naked foods because they provide empty calories.

Although moderate consumption of alcohol has some cardiovascular benefits, for people trying to lose weight it should not only be considered forbidden, taboo, prohibited and unauthorized, but it is also intoxicating. Since calories in alcohol are used (by your body) before stored fat calories, you don't tap into your present fat storage. Hence, it becomes very difficult to lose weight when you drink "socially." It has been found that people who are overweight or obese actually gain weight more easily when they drink alcohol.

Alcohol is a straight-to-the-stomach-and-hips kind of beverage. Calories from alcohol tend to be stored in the gut first. Because of its sugar content, it increases your blood sugar and subsequently your insulin levels. This starts the hunger cascade and before you know it, you are craving more sugar and junk foods. Is that why our local bar provides us with a menu full of unhealthy foods? We have a few drinks and then we ask for a menu.

Examples of Calories You Can Expect to Find in Favorite Alcoholic Drinks:

Wine calories, small glass; 125 ml

Red wine (85 cal.), Rose wine, medium (89 cal.), Sweet white wine (118 cal.), Dry white wine (83 cal.), Medium white wine (94 cal.), Champagne (80 cal.)

Beers, Lager and cider

Pint of lager (200 cal.), Pint of bitter (100 cal.), Pint of sweet cider (250 cal.), Pint of dry cider (200 cal.), Pale ale (91 cal.), Stout, bottled (105 cal.), Ordinary strength lager (85 cal.)

Spirits, one shot; 25ml

Vodka (50 cal.), Gin (50 cal.), Double shot of 90 proof (110 cal.), Whiskey (50 cal.), Southern Comfort (70 cal.)...Then add on additional empty calories for the drink mixer: Fizzy drink mixer (50 cal.), Baileys (80 cal.), Fruit juice mixer (50 cal.), Bloody Mary mix (115 cal.), Gin and tonic (171 cal.), Piña Colada (262 cal.), Whiskey sour (122 cal.),

And, of course, while you're relaxing with your favorite drink, you pack in the empty calorie snacks and foods: packed roasted nuts (300 cal.), packed salted nuts (250 cal.), and a large pizza (500 cal. per slice) or a burger (400 cal.).

The Journal of Clinical Investigation reported in 1999 that alcohol actually raises the level of blood free radicals. This puts oxidant stress on organs such as the heart and liver, and causes them to deteriorate. So there you have it, alcohol results in obesity yielding high blood pressure, high cholesterol, diabetes, heart disease, and also an excess of free radicals. The free radicals exacerbate all of these diseases and increase your aging process, which is why alcohol abusers always look older then they really are.

EXCESS ALCOHOL AND STRONG, HEALTHY BODIES CANNOT COEXIST!

Chapter Twelve

Agriculture and Technology

Read 5/13/09

"And every plant of the field before it was in the earth, and every herb of the field before it grew: for the Lord had not caused it to rain upon the earth, and there was not a man to till the ground."(Genesis 2:5 Holy Bible KJV).

"The Lord God took the man and put him in the Garden of Eden to work it and take care of it." (Genesis 2:15 Life Application Study Bible NIV).

As we know it, Africans had been eating a specific diet with vegetation as the foundation for nearly 6 million years. Because wild animal herds would flee from hunters to safety, as recent as a few thousand years ago, our ancestors developed an unnatural means of providing foods for the ravished masses; this marked the onset of the agricultural revolution. New plant foods were eaten and fed to both the humans and the newly tamed animals. The new science of cultivating soil, producing new crops and raising livestock was the

89

new way of doing things. It was also the end of eating to live longer and the beginning of a gamut of diseases. Human genes were designed by God to interact with certain foods and provide you a healthy strong body. Your genes, which are the map to proper bodily functioning, are very similar to those of your early ancestors. Your food choices have recently (just a few thousand years ago) changed and the result has become gene malfunctions that are incompatible with life.

With agriculture came the consumption of the mixtures of weeds (e.g. grains), drinking animal milk, unhealthy domesticated meats, and the addition of new and experimental foods to our diet. Things began to get even worse when, in the 1700s, the industrial revolution and industrialized, processed foods flourished. This was the marking of an era when the food industry began to refine food (e.g. whole grains and sugar) and feed it to the people. From this new way of doing things along with a considerable amount of greed stemmed fast food restaurants. This food caused even greater disarray to our genes.

As if the altered milk, grains and meat wasn't enough, man went even a step further and industrialized fats. This process was developed in the early 1900s and first commercialized in 1911 as a product very familiar to us; shortening. It all began when a German chemist by the name of Wilhelm Normann showed, in 1901, that liquid oils could be hydrogenated. He patented the process one year later then sold the rights to Normann's patent here in America. Then in 1911, the first hydrogenated shortening was marketed under the name Crisco. The shortening was composed largely of partially hydrogenated cottonseed oil and full of trans-fats. Further success came from the introduction of clever marketing tools such as free cookbooks filled with recipes that required the use of shortening. Since that time, shortening and other products mired down with trans-fats have become a mainstay in the African-American diet. In 1994, it was estimated that trans-fats contributed to 30,000 deaths annually in the U.S. from heart disease.

The transition from hunters and gathers to an agriculturally based society occurred without man knowing what effect it would have on our health. With agriculture came disease and despotism (a king or other ruler with absolute or unlimited power). The agricultural revolution began to spread like wild fire to all of the ends of the earth leaving only a few tribes of hunters and gatherers. The indigenous people of the Kalahari Desert are one of the few hunter-gatherer groups remaining. They are thought to be the oldest group of modern day man and even considered by some to be our "genetic Adam" tribe. They are a happy group of people who work fewer hours, sleep longer, have more leisure time and live less stressful lives than farming societies. The diet of these South Africans includes wild plants and animals which provides a better balance of vitamins and minerals as well as more protein. They don't concentrate on the high-carbohydrate crops (e.g. potatoes and rice) like the traditional farmers.

The first agricultural revolution is also called the Neolithic Revolution. It began about 8000-9000 years before the days of Christ. This era is associated with the adoption of early farming techniques and crop cultivation. The first agricultural revolution spurred major social changes, including a high population density, the organization of a hierarchical society, specialization in non-agricultural crafts, a standing army, barter and trade, and the expansion of man's "control" over nature.

Agriculture has forced people to live in very close proximity. This resulted in the spread of many diseases. Throughout the development of sedentary agricultural societies, disease spread more rapidly than it had during the time in which hunter-gatherer societies existed. The domestication of animals may explain the rise in deaths and sickness during the Neolithic Revolution from disease, as diseases jumped from the animal to the human population. Some examples of diseases spread from animals to humans are influenza, smallpox, and measles.

In his book entitled *The Worst Mistake in the History of Human Race*, Jared Diamond wrote:

"Hunter-gatherers practiced the most successful and longest-lasting lifestyle in human history. In contrast, we're still struggling with the mess into which agriculture has tumbled us, and it's unclear whether we can solve. Will we somehow achieve those seductive blessings that we imagine behind agriculture's glittering façade? Dr. Weston A. Price, an extremely intelligent and well respected dentist from Cleveland, Ohio was inquisitive enough to wonder what it was about our diets that made us unhealthy. His profound thinking led him to ask another question: 'Could it be our processed foods?' It was this type of thinking, in my opinion, that made him a genius. This is why he deserved the title The Charles Darwin of Nutrition and The Father of Preventive Dentistry."[1]

Food processing is the set of techniques and methods used to transform the raw ingredients of food substances into more attractive and marketable food for human consumption. Historically, various types of food processing existed during prehistoric ages with slaughtering, various styles of cooking (oven fires, smoking and steaming), fermenting, sun drying and preserving with salt. This was the extent of the advancement of food processing until the industrial revolution. Modern food processing technology was initially developed to serve the needs of military personnel. In the late 1700's, a candy maker, brewer, and baker by the name of Nicolas Appert developed a vacuum bottling process. He packaged his foods in bottles, corked them and submerged them in boiling water. The heat provided sterilization and prevented bacterial spoilage. In 1810, an Englishman named Peter Durand solved the problem of Appert's bottles breaking by storing them in tin-coated steel. Durand developed the "canister" with a soldered cover and this was the beginning of canned foods. In 1821, a canning plant was developed in Boston by William Underwood. Underwood canned a variety of goods: fruits, vegetables, and condiments. In 1862, Louis Pasteur developed pasteurization. Nearly a century later, Clarence Birdseye, after he noticed that fish and caribou meat exposed to Arctic air remained tender and fresh, developed his "Multiplate Quick Freeze Machine" and by 1925, he was in the frozen food business. Initially, he specialized in frozen fish fillets but later applied his quick freezing concept to meats, poultry, fruits, and vegetables.

Today, common food processing techniques include:

Spray drying, proofing, removal of unwanted outer layers, such as potato peeling or skinning of peaches, chopping or slicing (e.g. potato chips, diced carrots, or candied peels), mincing and macerating, emulsification, cooking by boiling, broiling, frying, steaming or grilling, mixing and the addition of gas such as air entrainment for bread or gasification of soft drinks.

Dr. Weston A. Price knew that food processing lowered the nutritional value of some foods, but was determined to prove to his peers how detrimental it was to his patients. Dr. Price traveled all over the world looking for the perfect group of indigenous people to study. He studied at least fourteen different cultures. And like most early day academicians, studying African people is where Dr. Price learned the difference between dietary perfections and imperfections. In 1935, his African voyage began in Mombassa, on the eastern coast of the continent. He next headed inland through Kenya to the Belgian Congo, then northward through Uganda and finally ended up in the Sudan.

His first realization was that the closer the African tribe's diet was to the original diet, the healthier the tribesmen. He found that they consumed more than four times the amount of water-soluble vitamins and minerals and at least ten times the amounts of fat-soluble vitamins as the diet of the more "civilized" people. From a dental standpoint, they would also have straight and strong teeth and strong and full jaws. In fact, he found six tribes that were completely free of dental decay. Dr. Price also recognized that those just one generation away from the original way of eating suffered from heart disease, cancer, narrowed faces, crowded teeth, weakened immune systems and a host of degenerative diseases.

He focused on one particular African tribe and gathered a host of confirmative information. The Dinkas, of the Sudan, were incontestably the healthiest tribe that Price studied. Their bodies, he explained, were in perfect condition and displayed great strength. Their diet consisted mostly of fermented whole grains, vegetables, fruit and fish. They ate very little to no red meat. Just as you probably suspect, they were without hypertension, diabetes, heart disease, cancers and other diseases that he found in the tribes that ate more similar to modern day man.

It is because of the impure thinking of the more recent farmers that we have been led into this day of dietary disaster and unhealthiness. On the other hand, it is people like Dr. Price and the word God that redirect us into a path of dietary dominance and longer lives. You, the reader and doer, will be the captain of the vessel to ensure that we get there.

Chapter Thirteen

Swine
(Not the other white meat)

The Lord says, "The end is near for those who purify themselves for pagan worship, who go in procession to sacred gardens, and who eat pork and mice and other disgusting foods. I know their thoughts and their deeds. I am coming to gather the people of all nations. When they come together, they will see what my power can do and will know that I am the one who punishes them." (Isaiah 66:17-19. Good News Bible, Good News Translation).

This is also detailed in verses 2:173, 5:3, 6:145, and 16:115 of the Qur'an. An exemplary ayat is quoted as:

"He has only forbidden you dead meat, and blood, and the flesh of swine, and any (food) over which the name of other than Allah has been invoked. But if one is forced by necessity, without wilful disobedience, nor transgressing due limits, then Allah is Oft-Forgiving, Most Merciful." (Qur'an).

People of various religions, especially Christians, time and time again debate over whether or not swine is an "unclean" and forbidden meat to eat. Like alcohol to an alcoholic or a casino to a gambling addict, pork is very tantalizing and a seemingly harmless product to African-Americans. This again proves that man seems to be attracted to things that are not good for him. "There is nothing like a bacon egg and cheese sandwich in the morning," I have been often told by friends of mine that I have challenged to stop eating pork. Another common response is: "if God didn't want man to eat swine, He wouldn't have made the pig." They obviously don't know that the pig has a specific purpose and it is not to be food for man.

It is considered unclean because God's Law deemed it so. God said that His word would not return void and we know that He is the same God yesterday, today and will be tomorrow. Many forget that animals were classified as "unclean" and "clean" well before the days of Judaism, Moses, Mosaic and Qur'anic laws, and the teachings of Jesus. Early man knew of unclean meats and did not partake of them. In the Old Testament, these aged laws of eating were simply a reminder or a reiteration to the Israelites since they were away from such practices while under bondage in Egypt. Therefore, these laws of eating were already given to mankind, but Israel was simply being reminded of them. We know this because in Genesis (7:2), God commanded Noah to take 7 pairs of the "clean" animals and 2 pairs of the "unclean" animals. At this point, Judaism did not yet exist and Moses had not been born. Furthermore, Jesus said that he came not to destroy the law but to fulfill the law (Mathew 5:17). Therefore, I charge naysayers to prove to me that Jesus ate pork since the Bible says that it is an unclean food. Nonetheless and regardless of your beliefs, you need to have a full understanding of how detrimental this meat product is to your health. Especially since you won't take the advice of your Holy Book.

Pork is often referred to as the other white meat. It is my opinion that marketers promote it as a white meat to imply that it is healthy since Americans

102

are buying less of it each year. Calling it the other white meat is simply a form of "suggestive" advertising. With the increase in our Muslim population and African-American's awareness of this unhealthy eating, we are putting less of this unhealthy meat on our plates and between our bread.

Pork is the only meat that is eaten all day long. Beef, fish, chicken, lamb and seafood are usually eaten only at lunch or dinner, but pork is "enjoyed" at breakfast, lunch and dinner. I ask you, who is in control, us or the pork we savor everyday and all day long? Just like slaves, pigs are slaughtered under cruel and unclean conditions. This is yet another reason why it should not be consumed.

Forbidden to you are carrion, blood, the flesh of swine, what has been hallowed to other than God, the beast strangled, the beast beaten down, the beast fallen to death, the beast gored, and that devoured by beasts of prey- excepting that you have sacrificed duly – as also things sacrificed to idols, and partition by the divining arrows; that is ungodliness." (Qur'an 5:3).

Pork is *cured* so that it may last longer on the shelves of the grocery markets and in your refrigerator. This is done by a process that includes salting, smoking or aging the meat. The resultant is a meat high in fat and sodium. For example, a 3oz piece of pork can have over 1500 mg of sodium in it. The daily recommended amount of salt is 500 – 2400 mg. In my opinion, African-Americans should consume no more than 1000 mg of sodium per day if we intend to prevent or reduce our rate of hypertension, kidney failure and other sodium related illnesses. My rule of thumb is: *if you can taste salt in your food, then there is too much salt in it.*

To produce bacon, brine (salt water) is injected into pork belly; it is smoked and further cured. Bacon is very high in both saturated fat and sodium. Ham is produced from the pig's leg. It is often cured, sometimes smoked, or even injected with sugars. Ham can also be dry-cured; which is the process of drawing out moisture to intensify the color and hopefully the flavor of the meat.

The pig is a filthy animal to say the least. It eats any and everything it has access to. This includes non-edible garbage, feces, other pigs, and even decaying animal flesh. Its purpose is the same as animals that dwell on the bottom of waters; to clean.

It seems that the pig is more obedient than many of us as it does exactly what God created it to do. Man, on the other hand, wants to do his own thing. As a result of his assigned nondiscriminatory eating, the pig harbors many bacteria, viruses, toxins, parasites and chemicals detrimental to your health. This is why trichinosis is a disease tagged as a risk associated with the consumption of undercooked pork. With swine not being a part of the original African cuisine, early man had to have known that it was an unclean animal and therefore did not eat it. Remember, it became a part of our diet only because (as slaves) we had no other food to eat. If abolition took place in 1865, why are we still eating like slaves?

Jesus considered the pig "unclean" and "unhealthy" as well. When Jesus encountered a man possessed with many demons and ordered them to leave the man, they asked to be sent into the swine (Mark chapter 5). Not a chicken, a cow, a fish or lamb. With the scripture referring to the demons as "unclean spirits," it seems logical that these unclean demons chose unclean swine and Jesus permitted their entrance into it since he considered them both unclean. I find it amazing that some of us cannot safely deduce that Jesus looked negatively upon the swine as being unclean. If the swine was already clean, wouldn't Jesus have kept it clean? And maybe he would have even eaten it.

Processed swine such as bacon and sausages are preserved with a chemical called sodium nitrite. This is added to protect pork eaters from meat contaminated with Clostridium Botulinum. When infected, eating the pork can cause botulism which is a fatal form of food poisoning. On its own, sodium nitrite reacts at high temperatures with compounds in the swine to form carcinogens (cancer causing agents) called nitrosamines. So is this really worth eating pork?

Again, regardless of your faith or opinion, it is a well know fact that today's pork is unhealthy. It does more harm to us than good and should not be consumed unless we have nothing else to eat. In reference to the specifics highlighted in the book of Deuteronomy, the pig it is a splitter of the hoof, but since there is no cud; it is unclean. This scripture goes on to explain that we are not to eat it or even touch its carcass. Let's be obedient to God's direction, so that our days may be longer on this earth.

"The time has come for us to turn away from the things we know are destroying us as an individual and destroying us as a people." Minister Louis Farrakhan.

Chapter Fourteen

Hypertension and Salt-Sensitivity

"And Jesus went forth, and saw a great multitude and was moved with compassion toward them, and he healed their sick." (Mathew 14:14. Holy Bible, King James Version).

Hypertension (high blood pressure), the so-called "silent killer," affects nearly 50 million people in the United States. It is called the silent killer because those suffering from it cannot tell when it is not controlled or is making them sick. Often times, it's not until one experiences some type of catastrophic event (e.g. stroke, heart attack, kidney failure) that they are either diagnosed with high blood pressure or began to comply with their doctor's recommendations. When it affects African-Americans, it usually has an earlier onset, is more difficult to treat, destroys more vital organs and is more lethal (than when it affects non African-Americans). According to a University of Maryland cardiologist, Elijah Saunders, one African-American dies every hour from a hypertension related

108

illness.[1] It has been scientifically proven that the African-American's blood pressure rises with an increase in salt intake. What is of paramount importance is that the converse is also found to be true. That is, the blood pressure of African-Americans will also decrease with a reduction in salt intake. Hence, we are sensitive to the amount of salt found in our diet. This is true for those with hypertension and without hypertension. Too much salt also contributes to osteoporosis, kidney disease, cancer of the stomach and worsens asthma.

It appears that African-Americans retain sodium more easily than non African-Americans. That means that we should eat it less often than others. According to a paper published by R. M. Peters, RN and J. M. Flack MD entitled *Salt Sensitivity and Hypertension in African-Americans,* the finding of salt sensitivity is so prevalent that it is considered to be a "hallmark" of black hypertension, as salt sensitivity is "found in 73% of all African-American hypertensive patients."[2] This is probably a survival response inherited from our African forefathers. In my opinion, salt retention allowed the African to hold onto water to prevent dehydration while traveling the hot and dry desert land. Early man had to walk many miles at times before coming across a body of water. The same applies to the cactus plant for example, it is found in hot climates and its stems and leaves are thick in comparison to most plants. This thickness is stored water, air and other nutrients needed to handle the rainless climates.

Salt is a solute. That is, it is capable of being dissolved in water. In addition to that, when salt accumulates in tissues it pulls water with it. This build up of salt and water generates a pressure on to the blood vessels within the tissue. If this pressure is great upon the vessels, the result is high blood pressure.

Studies prove, time and time again, that when African-Americans eat a diet that is rich in fruit and vegetables, high in fiber, low in red meats and pork, they can control their blood pressure, lose weight and rid their bodies from many other diseases. The Center for Science in the Public Interest (CSPI) also realizes that "A diet high in salt (sodium

110

chloride) is a major cause of heart disease and stroke. Despite pressure from the government and other health experts over the last quarter-century to reduce salt consumption, Americans are consuming more-not-less-salt."[3]

We must take our bodies through a "process of elimination" when it comes to harmful chemicals such as salt. This process must begin with the realization that the recommended daily amount salt is reached, and sometimes exceeded, just by eating store bought foods. Adding additional salt to your food during cooking takes you over and into the "overdose" status. You must cut down and then eliminate extra salt. Do this by not eating the foods that are high in salt: Tomato juice, Bologna, Fish sticks, French fries, Salami, Bacon, Canned soups, Lunchmeats, Pickles, Soy sauce, Hotdogs, Salted peanuts, Fast food burgers, Salted popcorn, Potato chips, some bottled water and Soft drinks. Now you know why these foods are so tasty to you and your family, it's the salt!

African-Americans must look at salt as a drug capable of disrupting the progression and the prosperity of our community; just as cocaine, alcohol, marijuana, violence and improper education are doing. The process of eliminating salt from our diets must start with each individual African-American and his household by:

- ✓ Not buying salt (sodium chloride) or bringing it into the home.
- ✓ Always instructing the server to remove the salt shaker from the table when visiting restaurants.
- ✓ Thoroughly rinsing off the salt before eating canned vegetables.
- ✓ Not using salt substitutes unless instructed by your physician, because salt substitutes contain a high concentration of potassium, which can be deadly.
- ✓ Not adding salt to foods you are cooking.
- ✓ Seasoning foods with lemon, vinegar, pepper and other spices instead of salt.
- ✓ Reading the nutrition facts labels for the salt content before buying

canned, frozen foods and other processed or pre-made foods.

✓ Realizing that it will take time before you become accustomed to eating a salt-free healthy diet. Be patient and "let goodness get you through it," as my grandmother used to say.

Make sure that you look at the Nutrition Facts labels on food packages and know the deceiving terminology:

Sodium Free- a product that contains 5 milligrams or less of sodium per serving.

Very Low Sodium- a product that contains 35 milligrams or less of sodium per serving.

Low Sodium- a product that contains 140 milligrams or less of sodium per serving.

Chapter Fifteen

Vegetarianism

Then God said, "I give you every seed-bearing plant on the face of the whole earth and every tree that has fruit with seed in it. They will be yours for food. And to all the beasts of the earth and all the birds of the air and all the creatures that move on the ground – everything that has the breath of life in it – I give every green plant for food." And it was so. (Genesis 1:29-30. Holy Bible, New International Version (NIV)).

With time, I found myself saying: **My people perish because of the lack of knowledge** (Hosea 4:6. Good New Bible, Good News translation). We lack the knowledge of how the food we are eating is killing us. Back in Africa, we ate a mostly vegetarian diet. Meat (mammals; beef and pork) was almost never eaten. Poultry (birds; chicken and turkey) was eaten very rarely. And fish would be eaten more often but still only on occasion. If and when an animal was hunted and eaten, it was a very lean source of protein, unlike our modern day domesticated meat. But for the most part, Africans ate: onions, grains,

114

legumes, yams, greens, sorghum, watermelon, pumpkin, okra, eggplant, cucumber, garlic and very little fruit. Before slavery, plant food made up about 90 percent of the West African's diet. It was well known to our ancestors, and to modern day scientists, that humans were **not** initially designed to eat meat. Carnivorous (meat-eaters) animals have distinctive traits from non-carnivorous animals. Because meat decays quickly and causes harm if held in the body for long periods of time, meat eaters have very short and powerful digestive tracts. The intestinal tract of meat eaters is only about 3 times their body length. Meat eaters also have strong hydrochloric acid production in their stomach to digest meat, skin, bones and connective tissues. Also, meat-eating animals do not have sweat glands. They sleep in the daytime and hunt during the cool night hour. This could be God's way of preventing man and meat eaters from crossing paths. Instead of sweating through pores, they decrease their bodily temperatures through their tongues. The vegetarian animals (i.e. the horse) are active during hot sunny days, perspire through their skin, have well developed salivary glands to digest grains and fruit, and sleep at night. Meat eaters must be able to run fast to catch their prey, they need claws to grab, and they must have sharp elongated teeth to puncture flesh. These characteristics are the most distinctive traits possessed by meat eating animals. They DO NOT have flat back teeth (molars) like plant-eating animals have in order to grind their food.

Man's characteristics are very similar to animals that eat fruits, grains, vegetables and nuts but are very far removed from animals that eat meat. The human digestive tract is over 12 times the length of our body. The stomach acid we produce is much weaker than that produced by meat-eaters. Our saliva glands (within the mouth) are well developed and contain ptyalin for grain and fruit digestion. Most of us work in the day and sleep in the night. Of course, we have pores in our skin that serve to cool us down through perspiration when we are exposed to heat. And, we do not have powerful jaws that house sharp or pointed front teeth. Instead, we have flat back molars. Human beings and herbivorous animals have little mouths with proportionately small heads, unlike carnivores, whose big mouths are designed for grabbing, gripping, tearing, killing and dismembering prey. Lastly, some carnivores are capable of producing vitamin C inside of their bodies whereas non-carnivorous animals must get it from their diets.

According to Genesis 1:29-30, man was created and instructed to eat grains and fruit and not the flesh of any animals. The Bible goes on to read later in the book of Genesis (9:2-3, Good News Bible, Good News translation): "The fear and dread of you will fall upon all the beasts of the earth and all the birds of the air, upon every creature that moves along the ground, and upon all the fish of the sea; they are given into your hands. Everything that lives and moves will be food for you. Just as I gave you the green plants, I **now** give you everything to eat." According to the scripture, this is when man became meat eaters (carnivores). This non-vegetarian manner of eating became acceptable after Noah experienced the great flood. Could it be that he allowed man to eat animal flesh since it would take time for vegetation to re-grow after being destroyed by the waters? Animal flesh, since they were vegetarians (Genesis 1:30), was composed of substances found within the plant. But did God intend for us to continue to eat animal flesh after the plants returned?

Vegetarianism, in general, is the practice of not consuming meat (beef, pork, chicken, turkey, fish, and seafood) with or without the use of other animal-based produce, such as dairy products or eggs. However, there are various types or levels of vegetarianism, categorized as follows:

Diet Name	Meat	Dairy	Eggs
Veganism	No	No	No
Ovo Vegetarianism	No	No	Yes
Lacto vegetarianism	No	Yes	No
Lacto-ovo vegetarianism	No	Yes	yes

As far as *lacto-* (meaning "milk") *ovo* (meaning "egg") *vegetarianism* is concerned, this excludes ingredients under which an animal must have died to obtain the product, such as meat, meat broth, cheeses that use animal rennet, gelatin (from animal skin and connective tissue), sugars that are whitened with bone char (e.g. cane sugar, but not beet sugar) and alcohol clarified with gelatin or crushed shellfish and sturgeon. Simply stated, lacto-ovo vegetarians don't eat any meat, but do eat eggs, milk, and other dairy products (e.g. cheese, butter, and yogurt). Some people are just lacto-vegetarians; they eat dairy products, but not eggs. Others are ovo-vegetarians; they eat eggs, but no other animal foods. A vegan eats absolutely no animal products. Amazingly, many vegans are opposed to even eating honey.

Others classifications of vegetarianism include:

- *Pesco/pollo* vegetarianism (semi-vegetarianism, poultratarianism) – will only eat certain meats depending on the particular diet (pesco-fish, pollo-fowl). As one who eats limited animal flesh (only chicken, turkey and fish), I would be considered a pesco-pollo vegetarian.
- *Flexitarianism* – prefer to eat vegetarian food, but make exceptions.
- *Freeganism* – consume things that do not support the production of additional products.

There are even more variations in vegetarianism if you consider that some are dedicated to health enough to eat only "organically" grown foods. Others abstain from drugs like alcohol and caffeine, avoid certain preservatives and additives and always take supplemental vitamins, herbs and minerals. It delights me to see that many practice fasting and avoid processed foods.

Some of yesterday's "famous" vegetarians were Mahatma Gandhi, Leonardo da Vinci and Albert Einstein. By far, the first and most influential vegetarian in European history was the Greek philosopher Pythagoras. The Pythagorean diet came to mean an avoidance of the flesh of slaughtered animals. In fact, vegetarians in Europe used to be called "Pythagoreans." He opposed violent deaths of all living beings and had a desire to create a universal and absolute law including injunctions not to kill "living creatures," to abstain from "harsh-sounding bloodshed," and to "never eat meat." The Pythagorean diet officially changed its title to vegetarianism (in 1847) and the Vegetarian Society was subsequently established to continue this original way of eating.

Man's hominid ancestors (referring to early man who walked on two feet), all of African descent, ate vegetarian diets with the exception of the occasional insects and grubs (the thick wormlike larva of certain beetles and other insects). Many famous African-Americans still subscribe to this original way of eating. It seems like African-

American vegetarians are budding up everywhere. Erykah Badu, Russell Simmons, Angela Bassett, India Arie, Common, Andre 3000 of Outkast, Darius McCrary, Dexter King, Traci Bingham, Dick Gregory and the late Coretta Scott King. Black Vegetarian Societies have even been established in Georgia and Texas.

Even the so-called Hip-Hop generation is adopting the vegetarian way of life. The uplifting and socially cognizant Hip-Hop duo Dead Prez rapped: "*I don't eat no meat, no dairy, no sweets – only ripe vegetables, fresh fruit and whole wheat... lentil soup is mental fruit and ginger root is good for the yout – fresh veg-e-table with the mayatl stew. Sweet yam fries with the green calalloo,*" in their song entitled "Be Healthy."[1] Also, soul food restaurants, Kwanzaa celebrations and church gatherings are being advised to become more vegetarian friendly when planning their meals.

People become vegetarians for many reasons. These may include religious reasons (Hindu, Moslem, Buddist, Seventh Day Adventist), health motives, fads, economic constraints, or moral (against the killing of animals) rationales. According to a recent survey of African-American vegetarians, the top three reasons why we decide to eliminate meat from our diet include: [1]

1. Health (34%)
2. Ethical (14%)
3. Spiritual or religious (12%)

What are the health benefits of being a vegetarian?

Since vegetarianism has such a wide variety of dietary exchange, it is difficult for me to generalize about the pros and cons of a vegetarian diet. I can, however, list the results of studies done on vegetarianism and health. Please keep in mind that someone who is informed and regimented enough to resist meat is more likely to: avoid smoking cigarettes, avoid abusing alcohol, exercise, read nutrition facts labels, practice safe sex and live an overall healthier life.

When compared to non-vegetarians in the U.S., studies have shown that vegetarians have a lower incidence of:

- ❖ Heart disease
- ❖ Colon cancer
- ❖ Coronary artery disease
- ❖ High blood pressure
- ❖ High cholesterol
- ❖ Obesity
- ❖ Type 2 diabetes

This may be because vegetarians consume less total fat, less saturated fat and cholesterol, more fiber, more fruits and vegetables, no cigarettes and less alcohol. These results can be found in non-vegetarian populations if they learned how to eat and live longer.

Vegetarianism often ignites major criticisms when not done properly. Non meat eaters can be at a greater risk of being deficient of calories, protein, iron, vitamin D and vitamin B-12. These nutritional challenges are usually not a significant problem except with vitamin B-12. This is because this vitamin is made by bacteria, fungi and algae. It is found within animal foods since they frequently bear the bacteria that make the B-12.

The plant is in a perfect state. All animals need plants to survive. Only plants can produce their own food and because of this scientists refer to them as producers. Plants need energy to survive, just like animals, but they get their energy directly from the sun. They use a process called photosynthesis to make food. How can the atheist doubt the existence of God?

"The uncontrolled and inappropriate use of antibiotics is highly responsible for the development of new strains of antibiotic resistant bacteria. Overuse of antibiotics has been shown to weaken the body's natural immune system." (World Health Report 1996, World Health Organization).[2]

Penicillin was the first antibiotic discovered and has led to the birth of a very lucrative business known as the pharmaceutical industry. "Anti," in Greek, "against," and "bio" means "life." Put together it refers to a substance that is "against life." Over half of the antibiotics produced each year in America are not used to save the lives of infected humans, but instead are used on livestock and poultry. Meat producers use antibiotics to treat and prevent disease since most domesticated animals live in crowded and unclean conditions. These antibiotics are also used to promote faster growth among the animals. The detrimental aspect of the overuse of these chemicals is bacterial resistance. As meat eaters, the resistant bacterium is introduced into man (from the animal) and we too house bacteria that are resistant to present therapy. The pharmaceutical industry is "behind the wagon" when it comes to producing drugs that can affectively ward off disease in man.

In June 2003, the New York Times published an article entitled *McDonald's Asks Meat Industry to Cut Use of Antibiotics*.[3] McDonald's, the world's biggest purchaser of meat, asked their major meat suppliers to cut back on the antibiotics because of the overwhelming evidence that this contributed to antibiotic resistance in animals and with the bacteria that cause disease in humans. Although meat producers also add growth hormones to animal feed to create "giant sized animals," McDonald's decision only affected the growth-promoting antibiotics. McDonald's also asked its suppliers to reduce the usage of a cipro-like antibiotic since its resistance could affect the treatment of anthrax among humans.

Although I spend at least 28 days a year as a vegan and greatly appreciate its effects, my non-vegetarian eating can be just as healthy. As a pesco-pollo vegetarian the remaining 337 days, I strive to choose the healthiest (low fat, organic, non-fried) animal flesh as often as possible. Vegetarianism has its place in our diets but to what extent is solely dependent upon the individual and their current state of health. Regardless of what plan you decide, know that what you eat will either cause or cure disease.

"Therefore, if what I eat causes my brother to fall into sin, I will never eat meat again, so that I will not cause him to fall." (1 Corinthians 8:13, Holy Bible).

Chapter Sixteen

Water

"Water, not milk, does the body good." R.
Eadie MD

When the maker created the earth, He
made it more than 70% water. And
when the maker created man, He made
him more than 70% water as well. He
also made man's brain and blood to be
composed of more than 70% and 83%
water, respectively. Water was God's
gift to man to not only be used for our
consumption, but also for the plants and
animals to use. While it transports
thousands of things within it, it also
serves as a means of transportation for
man. It houses some of the smallest
organisms and up to some of the largest
mammals. Through its auto-regulated
evaporation system, it is able to spread
itself across the earth for all living things
to enjoy. Water is the body's most
important nutrient, the only true thirst
quencher and the cure for many
diseases. Jesus was baptized in it,
walked atop it and changed it into wine.

The water molecule is composed of two hydrogen and one oxygen atom and has the divine capability of being in the gaseous, liquid or solid state. The importance of this element, to the human body, can never be stressed enough. It is amazing how the dairy industry has billboards throughout urban America proclaiming cow's milk to be an essential liquid and a cure all drink, yet water gets no publicity. It is water that helps remove the dangerous toxins that our bodies inhale, ingest (eating), and are exposed to via the hair and skin products we use. Water also cushions our joints, helps carry oxygen and nutrients into our cells and helps regulate body temperature.

In my practice, it bothers me to hear patients say they have trouble drinking the 64 ounces of water I advise. Look at it this way, while the 64 ounces that I recommend is certainly enough, some literature suggest drinking as much as half (in ounces) of your body weight. So, the 200 pound patient would be expected to drink 100 ounces of water. Now, doesn't that makes the 64 ounces seem reasonable and do-able?

Water is needed to keep your body functioning normal. The lack of adequate water intake leads to dehydration. Dehydration in turn slows down the metabolism and promotes weight gain. Your blood pressure also lowers with a low total body water level. This promotes clot formation at your blood which could be deadly. Also, your organs will start to fail or function improperly. Constipation, dry skin, increased incidence of urinary tract infections and recurring headaches are some of the early signs of dehydration.

The flavor of water can be altered to a more enjoyable and satisfying savor. An old-fashioned yet still common preparation is adding lemon to water. The Africa-American inventor, John Thomas White, had lemon water in mind when he invented and patented the lemon squeezer in 1896. He obviously knew the benefits of drinking water and the enhanced rewards of adding lemon. Besides tasting good, lemon water provides the following health benefits:

- ❖ It is an excellent source of Vitamin C. An average size raw lemon provides over 50 milligrams of Vitamin C.
- ❖ Enhances the beauty of your skin.
- ❖ It aids in cleansing the kidney and the liver.
- ❖ It stimulates your gastrointestinal tract enhancing digestion and elimination. It is also a good remedy for both diarrhea and constipation.
- ❖ It helps eliminate gastrointestinal symptoms such as bloating, heartburn and belching.
- ❖ It serves as an antiseptic, helping to prevent infections from a host of germs.
- ❖ A good source of calcium, magnesium and potassium.
- ❖ Provides relief from cold and flu symptoms.

Bottled water can be found in nearly every convenience store, supermarket and vending machine across American. It comes in different variations, such as flavored, fizzy, carbonated, seltzer, ground, fluorinated, sterile, tap, soda water, club soda, tonic, natural spring water, well water, purified water, and mineral water. Municipal (tap) water is usually treated before being bottled.

You may be surprised to find out that the vast majority of bottled water sold is treated municipal water. Two very popular brands of bottled water are simply tap water that has undergone reverse osmosis. Ironically they are made from makers of soft drinks. I also recommend that you stay away from waters with added artificial flavors, caffeine, sugar, artificial sweeteners as well as sodium. Always check the Nutrition Facts Label before making your purchase and stay away from those containing sodium (sodium bicarbonate or sodium chloride).

Bottled water that has been treated by distillation, reverse osmosis, or other FDA approved processes may be considered "purified water." Make sure that the bottled water you purchase is packaged with an expiration date printed on it. Even if the water itself is pure, a plastic container may leak chemicals into the bottled water. Storing your bottled water in cool and dark places help reduce these untoward reactions. Remember that bottlers erroneously claim that bottled water can be used indefinitely if stored properly. If the original water bottled is not pure, especially if it contained biological contaminants, then the water quality will continue to degrade regardless of the storage container or conditions. Hence the presence of expiration dates.

Drinking plenty of water should be just as important to you as cashing your pay check and remembering your birthday. These few water rules, if followed, will help to ensure that you make water drinking a habit:

1. Always have a glass of water before leaving your home each day.
2. Always complete a glass of water before ordering from a restaurant menu.
3. Always drink at least one glass of water with each meal.
4. Always drink a glass of water before, during and after each workout.

5. Always drink a glass of water before and during the consumption of any alcoholic beverages.
6. Always complete your 64 ounces of water at least 4 hours before bedtime.

Chapter Seventeen

Sugar

"The most detrimental and commonly abused drug in America is not alcohol, tobacco, cocaine, marijuana, heroin or vicodin; it is sugar!" R. Eadie, MD

Did God intend for us to add sugar to our diet? In my opinion, the best way to answer this question is to look at the purpose of sugar, its sources, the different types and its effect on the human body. Six billion years ago, man did not add sugar to his diet. Why? Because today's unnatural, refined, processed and artificial sugars did not exist. Currently, the average American consumes about 3 pounds of sugar per week, so let's take a closer look and discover the truth about sugar.

The main energy source for the human body is sugar **(C2H20)** so it is obviously very important, but the key is consuming *natural* sugars. Where did Adam and Eve get their sugar? Let's look at the brilliance of almighty God. Remember that oxygen is a waste product of plants and a very important and essential substance to man. Conversely, carbon dioxide (C02) is a waste product of man yet a very important and essential substance to plants. Now remember that God created the sun and its energy rays activate the green leaves of plants. Once activated, plants are able to combine the already created water (H20) and carbon dioxide (C02). So when you have many water molecules; Hydrogens (H2) and Oxygens (0) combining with many carbon dioxide molecules; Carbons (C) and Oxygens (02) you get:

H+H+0+H+H+0 + C+0+0+C+0+0 =
C2H20 + H20 + 04

As you can see, this reaction produces sugar with water and lots of oxygen remaining for us to use. To consume God's natural sugar, we simply have to eat the plants or eat the animals that ate the plants (in moderation, of course). The system for obtaining this sugar energy has already been set up for us.

Some natural sugars are also found in fruit and dairy products. The type of sugar found in fruit is called fructose and the type of sugar found in milk (and other dairy products) is called lactose. Fruit sugar is the sweetest naturally occurring sugar we have, thank you God! Over 70% of the world's population is lactose intolerant or in other words cannot breakdown the sugar in milk (and other dairy products). This leads me, and many others, to believe that God didn't intend for man to consume it. It cannot be a part of God's natural system if it makes us sick. Take a second and think about it!

The only wild animal that suffers from tooth-decay is the honey bear. So it's got to be the honey causing this disease! Honey decays teeth much faster than table sugar. Honey is also a natural sugar but I placed it separate from the ones above as it is also considered to be a refined sugar. In other words, excess consumption is bad for you. Although is tastes great, it has the highest calorie content of all sugars and is known to increases blood serum fatty acids significantly.

The introduction of unnatural culinary sugar into our diet is where greed and evil come into play and result in disease. Because of the "unattractive" appearance of colored foods, Europeans began to "refine" them to change them to a white color. Now, let's take a look at what they came up with:

White refined sugar is presently the most commonly used type of sugar throughout the world. It is typically sold as granulated sugar and varies by the size of the sugar crystals. Refined sugar is made by dissolving raw sugar and then purifying it with phosphoric acid (a white viscous liquid), mixing it with carbon dioxide and calcium hydroxide, or by taking it through various filtration processes. It is then filtered through bone char or activated carbon to decolorize it even more.

Raw sugars are colored sugars (yellow to brown) that are derived from the juices of sugarcane. Once the sugar is boiled and the water evaporated, the remaining crystals are considered raw sugars. Now, once the washing, centrifuging, filtering and drying is applied, it is no longer filled with fiber, stalk and nutrients and must now be called "refined." While many companies attempt to market raw sugars as natural and healthy, the processing of the sugar causes it to become a food high in calories and without nutritional value.

Mill white sugar also called **plantation sugar**, or **superior sugar**, is white colored sugar (raw) that has simply been bleached with sulfur dioxide.

Blanco directo is white colored sugar (raw) that undergoes both phosphatation (with phosphoric acid) and calcium hydroxide. The resultant is a white sugar, hence the name Blanco.

It wasn't until the early 1900's that cardiovascular disease and cancer began to threaten the longevity of African-Americans. This was subsequent to the insertion of unnatural, refined and processed sugars into our diets. It came along with the industrial revolution. Consuming sugar causes an increase in blood sugar levels which in turn causes a release of insulin (from the pancreas) into the blood stream as well. Insulin's function is to decrease the rise of blood sugar levels. It does so by pushing the sugar from the blood stream into the muscles so that they can use it as energy. An excessive rise in insulin also prevents the release of growth hormones in your blood, which in turn depresses your immune system. A decreased immune system = DISEASE. To make matters even worse, the triggered release of insulin also promotes the storage of fat and elevates triglyceride levels. Both are greatly linked to cardiovascular disease. Eating unnatural sugars on a regular basis inevitably leads to asthma exacerbation, mood swings, personality disorders, mental illnesses, nervous system disorders, diabetes, overweight, obesity, heart disease, gall stones, high blood pressure and arthritis.

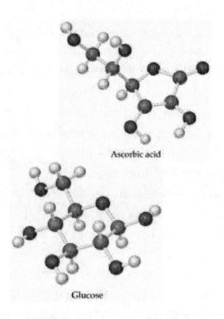

Ascorbic acid

Glucose

Vitamin C, as you probably know, helps your body fight off disease by strengthening your immune system cells. Since the 1970's, scientists have known about the link between vitamin C (ascorbic acid) and sugar (glucose). They are very similar in shape or in their chemical structure. In fact, almost all animals and some plants make their own vitamin C. The rat, mouse, hamster, cow, cat, dog, fox, and chicken can; whereas man, apes, guinea pigs, red-vented bulbul and the fruit eating bat cannot. All of the latter are vegetarian by nature. The human is the only one of these species who later began to eat meat. It will likely surprise you to learn that animals and plants can still produce vitamin C using natural sugars as the building block. It was Linus Pauling who first realized that your immune system cells (white blood cells) need high levels of vitamin C to fight off diseases. In the face of elevated blood sugar, he explained, they began to compete with one another to enter into the cells. The "door" entrance designed to let the vitamin C into the cell can also let the sugar in the cell since they are shaped similarly. The more sugar you have in your blood, the more sugar will get into your cells and the less vitamin C your cells have to use. There are four enzymes required to convert glucose into vitamin C. Man has the first three enzymes, having lost the fourth enzyme somewhere in evolution. Diabetics, please realize that even a blood sugar of 120 (mg/dL) will greatly reduce your immune system by not allowing the vitamin C to enter into your cells. Thousands of years ago in motherland Africa, losing the ability to produce vitamin C was not a major problem. Our ancestors lived in tropical regions where vitamin C containing food was abundant.

As far as your children are concerned, refined sugars interfere with their ability to learn and concentrate in school. And, although it has not been proven to cause ADHD, it certainly does worsen the symptoms. Parents must realize that sugar is more detrimental to children than adults. Properly metabolizing sugar requires a great deal of nutrients, but they have been stripped away from raw sugars. So during sugar metabolism these nutrients are stolen from a child's reserve which leads to their deficiency. This leads to other life-threatening diseases as well as overweight and obesity.

Childhood obesity is the new epidemic in this country and refined sugar is a major contributor. At least two out of every 5 children are currently overweight. This number has been predicted to double in the next 20 years. With the African-American child suffering the most, what are we doing to the future of our community?

Fruit juice has a high concentration of sugar and a lessened concentration of Vitamin C (because of the processing method) in comparison to fruit. It is therefore not nearly as healthy to give our children fruit juice in lieu of the actual fruit. They should be eating the fiber, vitamins and minerals that are present in the whole fruit and absent or significantly decreased in the juice. And now that we know how they compete at the cellular level because of their similar structures, we need much more Vitamin C present in our blood stream than sugar.

"Obese children now have diseases like type 2 diabetes, which used to occur only in adults. And overweight kids tend to become overweight adults, continuing to put them at greater risk for heart disease, high blood pressure and stroke. But perhaps more devastating to an overweight child than the health problems, is the social discrimination. Children who are teased a lot can develop low self-esteem and depression."[1]

Just as your body's healthy cells use sugar as its energy source, so does your body's unhealthy and cancerous cells. Anyone who has a diagnosis of cancer or even a family history of cancer will decrease their chances of surviving cancer if they eat refined sugar. Instead, they must learn how to eat and live longer. This will normalize your blood glucose, increase your immune system and allow your body to fight the disease.

Artificial Sweeteners

One thing that all living humans have in common is that they must eat food and drink water to continue to live. The spiritual "enemy" knows this to be true as well. What more efficient way to destroy the masses of people than through the food and water? All this adversary would need is a deceptive product that is used by almost everyone and in almost every type of food and his job can be accomplished with ease. Gathering a team to help deceive the masses by declaring this product safe would be another task but of little challenge. One product created to disrupt the health and longevity of man is the artificial sweeteners. With sugar being the most commonly drug abused in America, why not make a more detrimental but similar product. This creation can be paralleled to the transformation from powder cocaine to crack cocaine; similar chemical but more detrimental effects.

An artificial sweetener, also called a sugar substitute, is considered a food additive. They are used in foods to mimic the flavor of sugar (or corn syrup). They are often divided into two types: **non-caloric and sugar alcohols**. Both of which have a marketable advantage of adding very few calories and are often sweeter than table sugar. The four major sweeteners on the market are: aspartame, sucralose, saccharin and acesulfame.

Aspartame

I consider Aspartame, otherwise known as "Equal," "Spoonful" and "NutraSweet," as the worst of all of the artificial sweetener evils. Although it is 200 times sweeter than table sugar, it is affiliated with the biggest food fraud and trickery known to man. It is used in over 9,000 food products worldwide and consumed by over 200 million people in the United States. Unfortunately, this number probably includes you and your loved ones.

Aspartame = Phenylalanine + Aspartic Acid + Methanol

Aspartame is composed of two amino acids (L-phenylalanine and L-aspartic acid) plus methanol. Once eaten by a human, aspartame is broken down into both amino acids and methanol. Phenylketonuria (PKU), and the other causes of elevated blood phenylalanine, affect about one of every 10,000 to 20,000 Caucasian or Asian births. PKU is a genetic disorder in which the body lacks the enzyme needed to breakdown phenylalanine to tyrosine (another amino acid). Without treatment, the disorder can cause brain damage and progressive mental retardation as a result of the accumulation of phenylalanine and its breakdown products. This is why your diet drinks always list warning statements to phenylketonurics on its can or bottle. The incidence of PKU in African-

Americans is slightly less. These disorders are equally frequent in males and females.

The aspartic acid, like monosodium glutamate (MSG), is an excitotoxin. An excitotoxin is a harmful chemical that over excites or stimulates nerves within the brain and throughout the rest of your body. This increased arousal causes cellular death. During childhood development, the use of excitotoxins can lead to ADHD, learning disabilities, aggression, endocrine problems, infertility, premature puberty and menstrual difficulties. When used in adults, the result can be Parkinson's disease, Alzheimer's disease, ALS (Lou Gehrig's disease), Huntington's disease, cancers, and many other disabling illnesses.

Methanol is a colorless, poisonous, and flammable liquid. It is used for making paint strippers, carburetor cleaners for your automobile's engine and gasoline additives (methyl t-butyl ether). As an emergency room physician, it is important that I keep my clinical suspicions high since methanol causes drunkenness and blindness. The methanol is broken down into formaldehyde (embalming fluid) which is a cancer causing agent and very toxic. It is also metabolized into formic acid and DKP (diketopiperazine).

Today, hundreds of millions of U.S. citizens consume foods and drinks laced with this poison. It, like all demonic forces, comes in many different forms (children's vitamins, cakes, chewing gum, puddings, gelatins, diet soft drinks, etc).

If to you the dangers of using aspartame aren't obvious and the dangers of aspartame don't frighten you into abstinence, then at least help protect the children from such destruction.

Sucralose

If you were to look up the definition for Chlorocarbons, you would appreciate it to simply be a chemical compound containing carbon and chlorine. And, you would find chlorine defined as a nonmetallic element belonging to the halogens; best known as a heavy yellow irritating toxic gas; used to purify water and as a bleaching agent and disinfectant. Its chemical symbol is *Cl.* Chlorocarbons have been known for years to cause organ genetic and reproductive damage. As indicated in its definition, chlorine is a highly poisoning agent. It is irritating to the respiratory tract and depletes the body of vitamin E. As you are probably guessing by the mere title of this section, Sucralose (sold under the name Splenda) is a Chlorocarbon. It's chemical structure includes three chlorine (Cl) atoms.

Sucralose was discovered in 1976 by British researches employed by Tate & Lyle Ltd, a sugar refinery. Splenda is a non-caloric artificial sweetener that is actually 600 times sweeter than table sugar (sucrose). It wasn't until Tate & Lyle teamed with Johnson & Johnson forming McNeil Specialty Products Company that Splenda was made commercial. In 1988, the Food and Drug Administration approved Splenda to be used in a variety of food products. Diet RC cola was the first to contain Splenda in that same year.

Sucralose is made by chlorinating white sugar (sucrose). The chemical structure of sucrose is disfigured after three chlorine *(Cl)* atoms replace three hydroxyl *(OH)* groups.

The U.S. Food and Drug Administration revealed that Splenda has been shown to shrink the thymus gland of humans by 40%. Now, how important is the thymus gland? The thymus gland is the major gland in your immune system. It is responsible for producing your T Cells, the very cells that are destroyed by the Human Immuno-deficiency Virus (HIV). It also causes swelling and calcification of the kidney and enlargement of the liver. Splenda users may experience cancers, reduced growth rates, diarrhea, spontaneous abortions and anemia as well.

Under normal circumstances, your hunger center knows when to tell you to stop eating. This appetite control is lost with the consumption of artificial sweetener. Some studies even show that NutraSweet actually increases ones appetite. There just isn't anything positive I can share with you about using artificial sweeteners.

Sugar Alcohols

The last time you ate something that claimed to be "sugar free" or had "no sugar added," but had the sweet taste probably also had hidden calories that came from sugar alcohols. Don't worry, sugar alcohols don't intoxicate you, they are called so because part of their chemical structures resemble sugars while the other part of their structure resembles alcohols. Unlike artificial sweeteners, they occur naturally in foods and are actually extracted from plant products such as berries and fruits. They are converted into glucose like other foods, however it occurs very slowly. This means that your blood insulin response will occur much slower, which is ideal for diabetics. Sugar alcohols are a much healthier choice than artificial sweeteners.

It should be very obvious now how important it is for you to familiarize yourself with Nutrition Facts Labels. Then, and only then, will you really know what you're putting into your body. Common sugar alcohols are mannitol, sorbitol, xylitol, lactitol, isomalt, maltitol and hydrogenated starch hydrolysates.

Under normal circumstances, carbohydrates (e.g. table sugar) contain 4 calories per gram. Traditional artificial sweeteners, such as Splenda, contain no carbohydrates and therefore provide zero calories. On the other hand, sugar alcohols contain about 2.6 calories per gram. They are ideal for chewing gums since they do not cause tooth decay like sugar does.

Xylitol is naturally found in fruit, vegetables, cereals, mushrooms, straw, corncobs and some cereal. Xylitol has the same degree of sweetness as sugar. Xylitol is also called "wood sugar."

Mannitol occurs naturally in sweet potatoes, pineapples, olives, carrots, and asparagus. Food manufactures extract Mannitol from seaweed. It only has about 60% of the sweetness found in table sugar so more of it must be used. It is known to cause bloating and diarrhea because of the extended period of time it stays in your intestines.

Sorbitol is also found naturally in fruits and vegetables. It is manufactured from corn syrup. It has close to 50% of the relative sweetness of sugar. It is less likely to cause bloating and diarrhea than Mannitol. It is also used in sugar-free gums and candies.

Lactitol is a favorite for manufactures of sugar-free ice cream, chocolate, hard and soft candies, baked goods, sugar-reduced preserves and chewing gums. It has about 35% of sugar's sweet taste.

Hydrogenated starch hydrolysates (HSH) are produced by the partial hydrolysis of corn. They can have up to 90% of a sugary influence. You may notice these listed on the nutrition facts labels of mouthwashes.

Maltitol is nearly 75% as sweet as sugar. This sugar alcohol is what gives the creamy texture in many creamy foods such as ice creams and desserts.

Isomalt is about 55% as sweet as sugar and holds its sweetness even when exposed to heat. It is often used in lollipops, cough drops, hard candies and toffee.

Chapter Eighteen

The United States Government and our Diet

"Then Peter and all the other disciples answered and said, we ought to obey God rather than man."
Acts 5:29

"The king assigned them a daily amount of food and wine from the king's table. They were to be trained for three years, and after that they were to enter the king's service...But Daniel resolved not to defile himself with the royal food and wine, and he asked the chief official for permission not to defile himself this way...At the end of the ten days they looked healthier and better nourished than any of the young men who ate the royal food. So the guard took away their choice food and the wine they were to drink and gave them vegetables instead. To these four young men God gave knowledge and understanding of all kinds of literature and learning. And Daniel could understand visions and

dreams of all kinds." Daniel 1: 5, 8,
15-17.

The United States Government has been
regulating our food and advising us on
what to eat for over 100 years yet we are
becoming an unhealthier group of
people. Could this be because we are
listening to the urgings of man instead
of obeying the word of God? In 1862,
President Abraham Lincoln founded the
United States Department of
Agriculture and its United States Bureau
of Chemistry. With the fast growing
meat packing industry and the import
of animals, new diseases began to show
up the in blood of Americans. In 1865,
not only was slavery abolished and
President Abraham Lincoln
assassinated, but that same year
Secretary Isaac Newton urged congress
to enact legislation to quarantine these
imported animals to prevent the spread
of disease but not much was
accomplished. It wasn't until 1905 after
Upton Sinclair wrote a novel titled "The
Jungle" which exposed the inhumane
and filthy behaviors of Chicago
meatpacking workers that the U.S.
government took action. In 1906,
President Theodore Roosevelt passed

the Food and Drug Act and the Meat Inspection Act. The USDA's Bureau of Chemistry later was renamed the Food and Drug Administration. This particular branch is now called the Department of Health and Human Services. In the 1960's the onset and rise in heart disease gave the USDA reason to wonder if the foods they approved for us to eat were killing us. The Government began to make dietary recommendations and objectives for its citizens. The "basic four" (milk, meats, fruits, vegetables and grains) seemed to be giving us nothing but an increase in weight, strokes and heart attacks. In the 1970's, the USDA then added a fifth category to the Basic Four: fats, sweets and alcoholic beverages and then recommended that they be consumed in moderation.

Finally in 1977, the United States Senate Committee on Human Needs and Nutrition published *The Dietary Goals for the United States*. This publication did an excellent job at linking these new major illnesses directly to the food we were eating. To help decrease the rate and incidence of these killer diseases, the committee recommended several changes in the American diet. They suggested an increase in the consumption of fruits, vegetables and whole grains, while decreasing the intake of sugars, salts, fat, cholesterol and meat. The document stated:

> The simple fact is that our diets have changed radically within the last 50 years, with great and often very harmful effects on our health. These dietary changes represent as great a threat to public health as smoking. Too much fat, too much sugar or salt, can be and are linked directly to heart disease, cancer, obesity, and stroke, among other killer diseases. In all, six of the ten leading causes of death in the United States have been linked to our diet.

The publication went on to state:

> The diet of the American people has become increasingly rich – rich in meat, other sources of saturated fat and cholesterol, and in sugar ... We might be better able to tolerate this diet if we

were much more active physically, but we are a sedentary people ... It should be emphasized that this diet which affluent people generally consume is everywhere associated with a similar disease pattern – high rates of ischemic heart disease, certain forms of cancer, diabetes and obesity...

The over-consumption of fat, generally, and saturated fat in particular, as well as cholesterol, sugar, salt and alcohol have been related to six of the ten leading causes of death: heart disease, cancer, stroke, diabetes, arteriosclerosis and cirrhosis of the liver.[1]

There is no evidence to suggest that mandates were put in place to ensure that we took heed to the Senate Committee's recommendations. Things have only gotten worse since this was released in 1977, a time before the spread of fast-food restaurants, videogames, microwaves and other contributors to unhealthy living.

In the 1980's, in an attempt to begin improving the health and diet of Americans, the USDA began using an African symbol, one of the wonders of our world, to encourage a change in dietary habits, by introducing the food pyramid. Unfortunately, this 'novel' idea only exacerbated the problem. The food pyramid was constructed to express three main ideas: variety, proportionality and moderation. It was finally released in 1992 and was thought to be even more eater-friendly when the 1994 Nutrition Labeling and Education Act forced all grocery store foods to carry a nutritional label. The information provided by the food pyramid suggested things differently than the United States Senate Committee on Human Needs and Nutrition. It recommended 2-3 servings per day of foods from the milk, yogurt and cheese group as well as from the meat, poultry and fish group. It didn't take in consideration the variety of cultures and their respective foods. And, according to a Harvard University scientist Dr. Walter Willett, this food pyramid was not even up-to-date with the current nutritional research. Obesity in our children soon resulted from school lunch programs and parents following these recommendations. It misled people by suggesting that all fats are bad, all complex carbohydrates were good, meat (animal) proteins were good, dairy products are essential, and potatoes were healthy. It also failed to mention the importance of daily exercise and the health benefits of taking daily multivitamins. Not only was the pyramid ineffective in establishing healthy guidelines for Americans in general, but it certainly was not designed with the descendants of African people in mind. In fact, it was not designed for any human being. The goal to eradicate food induced illnesses was not accomplished as planned.

*"In that day there will be **an altar** to the Lord in the heart of Egypt, and a **monument** to the Lord at its border. It will be a **sign and witness** to the Lord Almighty in the land of Egypt." (Isaiah 19:19 - 20. Holy Bible, King James Version).*

African-Americans are descendants of the world's most intelligent people. From the first advanced civilization (Egypt), to the father of medicine (Imhotep) and up to the first wonder of the world (the pyramid). A group of three pyramids, Khufu, Khafra, and Menkaura located at Giza, Egypt, outside modern Cairo, is often called the first wonder of the world. The pyramid has always represented intelligence, strength and deep mysteries that only our forefathers understood. It was even well respected by our Masonic founding fathers, who used it to represent the great seal of this country.

Then again, in 1992, the U.S. government borrowed the symbol to represent "healthy" eating. The base of the food pyramid listed the foods we are to eat more of and most often. The apex of the pyramid lists foods we are to eat few of and less frequently. For example, at the base one would find breads, cereals, rice and pasta with 6 – 11 servings recommended daily. The next level of the pyramid included the vegetable (3 – 5 servings) and fruit (2 – 4 servings) groups. Next, the dairy (2 – 3 servings) and a larger group including meats, eggs, nuts and dry beans (2 – 3 servings). Finally, Fats, oils and sweets are at the apex so should be eaten sparingly.

These recommendations have contributed to the failing health of Americans. The Physician's Committee for Responsible Medicine published an article entitled, "Dietary Guidelines for Americans 2000 The Politics of Food: A Brief History of the U.S. Dietary Guidelines," which suggested that the original food pyramid was influenced by the meat and dairy industry to increase the sales of their products.

For African-Americans, this plan was never conducive to a long and healthy life for several reasons:

1. **The pyramid is not genetic or culture sensitive**. For example, milk and dairy products carry a milk sugar called lactase. African-Americans, like the majority of the world, stop producing the enzyme lactase (which helps our bodies process the sugar lactose) at an early age, soon after we are weaned off of our mother's breast milk. Without the lactase enzyme, our bodies are unable to properly process the sugar lactose and we experience nausea, bloating, excessive gas,

diarrhea, abdominal cramps and other unpleasant symptoms. The food pyramid also did not take into consideration our body's response to this new way of eating since our journey from Africa. Our bodies were used to eating many raw fruit and vegetables, increased fiber and little to no meat.

2. **The pyramid lists ALL fats at the apex**. This insinuates that fats should rarely or almost never be eaten. The thought that "a fat is fat" is inaccurate. It is true that fats such as those that are **saturated or trans** are bad for your health and are proven to clog arteries causing heart disease and stroke. However, to suggest that we are to avoid ALL fats is inaccurate and unfair advice since good fat is absolutely essential for good health. Our bodies need both polyunsaturated and monounsaturated fats for the following reasons:

1. Fat is a concentrated source of stored energy.
2. Essential fatty acids support heart health, building a strong immune system and boosting metabolism.
3. Fat keeps your blood and body warm and protects internal organs.
4. Fat is needed for the transport of fat-soluble vitamins (E, A, D & K) throughout the body.
5. Some fats are used by your body for hormonal production and neurological communication.

3. **The pyramid doesn't consider the overweight or obese patients**. The treatment of overweight and obesity starts with education. This is the only sure way to prevent recurrence of these diseases. In most cases, the treatment plan must include a reduction in the daily caloric intake. After all, one pound is

equal to 3,500 calories. The food pyramid doesn't recommend a specific number of calories, mention how important it is to maintain a normal BMI, point out the risks of alcohol use or promote daily vitamin use.

4. **The pyramid suggests that ALL carbohydrates are good and for everyone**. Just like fats, there are allies and enemies in the world of carbohydrates. The food pyramid makes no mention of this, nor does it even attempt to explain the important difference between **simple** and **complex** carbohydrates. Simple carbohydrates are simple sugar foods such as chips, cookies, candy and crackers. Six to eleven servings per day of any of these could lead to becoming overweight or obese. Complex carbohydrates are the type we should be eating. Complex carbohydrates should come from whole grain foods that are high in fiber, such as whole grain breads.

5. **The pyramid doesn't consider salt sensitivity**. Like lactose intolerance, a significant amount of people have blood pressure elevations and water retention after consuming foods high in salt. This should be highlighted and salt reduction should be recommended.

A simplified, yet ideal food pyramid for African-Americans to follow would be:

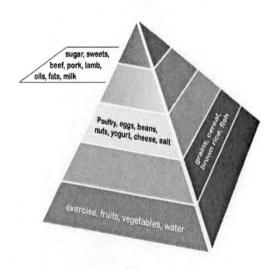

Remember, items at the top (sugar, sweets, beef, pork, lamb, oils, fat & milk)

should be consumed less frequently and those at the base of the pyramid should be consumed more often.

Chapter Nineteen

Permissible and Forbidden Meats

"And the flesh of living beings is not all the same kind of flesh; human beings have one kind of flesh; beasts another; birds another; and fish another."(1 Corinthians 15: 39. Good News Bible, Good News Translation).

If cleanliness is next to Godliness, then certainly "clean" and "unclean" foods must be discussed. Your opinion about this matter may depend upon the following: your cultural influences, your level of medical or scientific education, your teachings as a Christian, your conviction in Judaism and your belief in Islam. Some Christians refer to the book of Leviticus and Deuteronomy for instructions on what meats they should or should not eat. Other Christians believe that all meats are considered clean since the new covenant or New Testament. As a Christian and the author of this book, I am at liberty to express my view point on such a matter so please bear with me.

I have spent several hours of my free time lecturing to high school students about abstinence. The reality of sexuality on the high school level is that it exists much more than parents would like to believe. Therefore, I often end my lectures with the popular saying, "whenever you have sex, remember that you are having sex with all of your partners' previous partners as well." That is the same concept I use to decide what meats are good for me. This primary concept, I believe, comes from God's instructions on dietary's laws. Many of the animals that God declared forbidden are scavengers who eat other animals. If these scavengers eat contaminated meat, those who eat the scavenger meat will also become contaminated. Thus, God doesn't want us to eat the scavenger. Also, I believe God would like for us to consume animals that thoroughly digest the foods they eat. For that reason, he has instructed (Leviticus 11:3; Deuteronomy 14:6) us to eat animals that chew their cud (semi-digested food). These animals actually have four parts to their stomach. The first two chambers provide some digestion to the food. They then regurgitate (vomit) the food and then re-swallow it again into the next two chambers for additional digestion. This eliminates more of the impurities and provides for a healthier animal. Other "unclean" foods are animals that would kill and eat human beings, eat the waste products of other animals or are not intended to provide nutritious benefits. In terms of fish, God instructed (Leviticus 9-12) us to eat those with fins and scales. It is in my opinion that these fish were allowed because they were the least likely fish to be contaminated while being sought after as prey. The scales serve as protectors and make it difficult to puncture the flesh of these fish during attacks. The fins allow the fish to move quickly and maintain stability while swimming away from prey. Thus, reducing the exposure to contaminants such as bacteria, viruses, fungi, etc. from the teeth/mouths of unclean animals (or fish) attempting to eat them. The scales and fins also allow the fish to swim at the upper vastness of the waters where it is more pure or less contaminated.

I believe that God is the same God yesterday, today and tomorrow. To be precise, He was the same God in the Old Testament as He is in the New Testament. Anything else, I believe, is a misinterpretation of the scripture and would be unfair to man. Even more, if you examine the "unclean" foods logically, you can appreciate the scientifically proven disadvantages of consuming such meats. Consider the works of Dr. David I. Macht and how his studies proved Old Testament "clean" meats to be less toxic than the listed "unclean" meats. Or, how the works of Dr. J. M. Flack revealed the fact that foods with high salt concentrations cause hypertension in African-Americans.[1] At the end of the day, I believe whether you declare meat clean, kosher or halal, God will allow you to use what you have as long as you use it for the vindication of His name.

"If you obey my laws, my commands and my decrees...I will keep you free from every disease" (Deuteronomy 7:11-15. Holy Bible, King James Version). Now that should be all I have to remind you of, but I will continue. Is it Godly, intelligent, or even advisable to eat

foods that you know will cause you harm? Would you take penicillin for a bacterial infection knowing that you have an allergy to it? Your goal should be to prevent yourself from experiencing the diseases that plague your ancestors and family members such as colon cancer, heart attacks and strokes.

It is always reassuring to learn that many of the animals we eat are considered to be clean. The animals that chew the cud and are considered clean are: antelope, bison (buffalo), caribou, cattle (beef, veal), deer (venison), elk, gazelle, giraffe, goat, hart, ibex, moose, ox, reindeer and sheep (lamb, mutton). The fish with fins and scales that are considered clean are: anchovy, barracuda, bass, black pomfret (or monchong), bluefish, bluegill, carp, cod, crapple, drum, flounder, grouper, grunt, haddock, hake, halibut, hardhead, herring (or alewife), kingfish, mackerel, mahi-mahi (or dorado), dolphin fish, smelt (or frost fish or ice fish), snapper (or ebu, job fish, lehi, onaga, opakapaka or uku), sole, steelhead, sucker, sunfish, tarpon, trout (or weakfish), tuna (or ahi, aku, albacore, bonito, or tombo) and whitefish. The birds considered to be clean include: chicken, dove, duck, goose, grouse, guinea fowl, partridge, peafowl, pheasant, pigeon, prairie chicken, ptarmigan, quail, sagehen, sparrow (and other songbirds), swan, teal and turkey.

More importantly, we must familiarize ourselves with the animals that are considered to be unclean. Animals with unclean characteristics include: swine (boar, peccary, pig, pork, hog, bacon, lard, pepperoni and most sausage), canines (coyote, dog, fox, hyena, jackal, wolf), felines (cat, cheetah, leopard, lion, panther, tiger), equines (ass, donkey, horse, mule, onager, zebra), armadillo, badger, bear, beaver, camel, elephant, gorilla, groundhog, hare, hippopotamus, kangaroo, Llama, mole, monkey, mouse, muskrat, opossum, porcupine, rabbit, raccoon, rat, rhinoceros, skunk, slug, snail, squirrel, wallaby, weasel, wolverine, worm, and all the insects except those in the locust family. The marine animals without scales and fins that are considered to be taboo include: bullhead, catfish, eel, European, turbot, marlin, paddlefish, sculpin, shark, stickleback, squid, sturgeon (includes caviar) and swordfish. The shellfish that are unclean include: abalone, clam, crab, crayfish, lobster, mussel, prawn, oyster, scallop and shrimp. The soft body aquatic animals that are forbidden include: cuttlefish, jellyfish, limpet, octopus and squid (calamari). The sea mammals that we are not to eat include: dolphin, otter, porpoise, seal, walrus and whale. The birds of prey and those that are scavengers that are considered unclean include: albatross, bat, buzzard, condor, coot, cormorant, crane, crow, cuckoo, eagle, flamingo, grebe, grosbeak, gull, hawk, heron, kite, lapwing, loon, magpie, osprey, ostrich, owl, parrot, pelican, penguin, plover, rail, raven, roadrunner, sandpiper, seagull, stork, swallow, swift, vulture, water hen and woodpecker. We should not eat many of the reptiles (alligator, caiman, crocodile, lizard, snake and turtle) and amphibians (blindworm, frog, newt, salamander, toad) either.

Many Christian leaders negate the need to follow these biblical laws since they came under the old covenant. This covenant, some are taught, began with Abraham and the Israelites and ended with the new covenant. They go on to remind us that "You are free to eat anything sold in the meat market, without asking any questions because of your conscience," as it is written in 1 Corinthians 10:25. Let us also be reminded that thousands of years before the birth of Abraham, the covenant and the nation of Israel, God had already declared certain foods as "clean" and "unclean." Actually, even in the beginning with Adam and Eve, He considered certain foods permissible and forbidden. Meat wasn't mentioned since man was a vegan during those times. Fast-forwarding biblical history to the time of Noah, Genesis 7:2 reminds us that He declared certain meat as clean and unclean. Notice, God didn't have to define clean and unclean foods to Noah as He had to do for Adam, Eve and the Israelites. This must mean that they were already aware of the differences between the two groups. And, there is no biblical evidence that God has changed, does change or will change. According to 1 Corinthians (Chapter 10:23), we are allowed to do anything. That may be true, but that "anything" may kill us.

Chapter Twenty

Fiber

"Then after all this, the Lord brought on the king a painful disease of the intestines. For almost two years it grew steadily worse until finally the king died in agony." (2 Chronicles 21:18-19. Good News Bible, Good News Translation).

Eating plenty of fiber on a daily basis for its benefits has been a well known practice among African people since the beginning of time. It wasn't until the works of Dr. Dennis Burkitt that the rest of the world began to appreciate this African wisdom. According to Dr. Burkitt, as long as the native Africans didn't eat foods similar to the visiting Europeans, they stayed very healthy. Dr. Burkitt was a well known and respected physician that visited Africa for over 20 years as an assignment for the British Navy. While caring for the British soldiers and their wives, he couldn't help but notice how they suffered from many chronic diseases that did not appear to affect the native Africans.

The British soldiers and their wives suffered from diseases such as: appendicitis, overweight, obesity, high cholesterol, appendix and gallbladder cancer, coronary heart disease, colon and rectal cancers, diverticulosis, diverticulitis and many other terrible illnesses. The major difference between the two groups of people was their diet. The British ate an animal-based diet with lots of refined sugars, white flour and less than 10 grams of fiber per day. On the other hand, the native Africans ate a plant-based diet that contained about 100 to 150 grams of fiber per day. From this, he immediately knew that the fiber was important and thus developed his research.

Knowing how fiber works, Burkitt's research compared the stools of the British and African people. His analysis revealed small compact stools among the British that took 72 to 100 hours before passage out of their bodies. The Africans' stool was much larger and heavier and passed effortlessly within 18 to 24 hours. Next, he found that when the Africans ate the foods that the British ate, they developed the ailments that were killing and causing them to suffer. Today, the African-American has stool transit times similar to the British since we have adopted the European way of eating. As a result, we now suffer more readily from gout, obesity, skin disorders, appendicitis, hemorrhoids, constipation, heart attacks, diverticulitis, type 2 diabetes, dental problems, irritable bowel syndrome, varicose veins, gall stones, ulcerative colitis, Crohn's disease, multiple sclerosis, hypertension, cardiovascular disease and kidney stones.

To call the early African people primitive is a misnomer. They should have been called advanced intellectuals. Based on the way we eat, today's descendents of Africans should be called primitive. Although modern recommendations are that we eat about 25 grams of fiber per day, our ancestors ate over 100 grams daily. We still seem to average less than 10 grams per day. Fiber is also associated with decreased hunger, therefore can help combat our adult and childhood obesity. Isn't it amazing how God has already provided the solution to many of our health problems? We need to get back to the basics and start eating more righteously so we can live longer!

Fiber is a coarse, indigestible plant matter, consisting primarily of polysaccharides such as cellulose, that when eaten, stimulate movement of your intestines. African-Americans often refer to fiber as "roughage" and in science they are called carbohydrates. Fiber is present in all plants that we eat for food (e.g. fruit, grains, legumes and vegetables).

Fiber can be classified into two types, soluble and insoluble. Soluble fiber partially dissolves in water whereas insoluble fiber does not. Examples of soluble fiber include oatmeal, nuts, legumes (dried peas, beans, lentils), pears, blueberries, strawberries, apples, nuts, seeds and oat bran, etc. Samples of insoluble fibers are whole wheat breads, barley, brown rice, wheat bran, carrots, zucchini, celery, cucumbers, etc.

Your Bible, in the book of Daniel (1:1-20), proves the concept that high fiber foods produce good health. Read how Daniel and other young, healthy, good looking and intelligent Israelite boys were chosen to serve in the royal court. King Jehoiakim ordered them to three years of special training. During this training, Ashpenaz was to teach them to read and write the Babylonian language and feed them the same food and wine as the royal court. Daniel made up his mind to eat like his ancestors and not of this new diet. He coaxed the guard into feeding him and his three friends nothing but vegetables and water for ten days and then to compare them to young men that were eating the food of the royal court. The servants who ate the King's foods after 10 days were unhealthy as opposed to Daniel and the other Israelites that ate the vegetables. They were healthier and had strong manly bodies. Eating foods high in fiber also provided development in "wisdom and understanding."

If the worldwide bestseller isn't enough to convince you to eat high fibrous food, perhaps the following excerpt from the *Townsend Letter for Doctors and Patients* (August-Sept, 2005) by Wayne Martin will:

"There was a most remarkable report in the January 1960 issue of the American Journal of Cardiology by Robert O'Neal et al. of Washington University School of Medicine about the black population of Uganda. In 1960 this population had no deaths from heart attacks, from myocardial infarction at all. I had an interview with Dr. O'Neal in 1961. He told of this population of Uganda. They were strict grain vegetarians and the grains were corn, millet and barley. They boiled their grains in clay pots.

This population was also free from colon cancer. An English doctor, Denis Burkett, was in Uganda in the 1960s and he took note of the high fiber content of their grain diet and he suggested that the high fiber was the cause of the freedom from colon cancer among them.

In a whole grain diet there is about 5 grams of linoleic acid which is acted on by the enzyme delta-6-desaturase to form gamma linolenic acid which made the very low content of arachidonic acid in the blood of these Ugandans even lower."[1]

It will help you to know that arachidonic acid is the building block of bad eicosanoids. Also of note is that it is an Omega-6 fatty acid. Arachidonic acid is metabolized to eicosanoids which are highly active in immune and inflammatory responses. It is also known to stimulate blood clotting.

Both heart disease and cancer appears to be the result of "bad" eicosanoids. Cancer is the result of controlled and accelerated production of these eicosanoids. They are located in the fatty tissue of muscle meat and organ meat. Maybe this is why the Bible warns us against eating the fat of animals. Bad eicosanoids are found in the eggs and milk of animals fed on grains. Therefore, be sure to eat only lean chicken breast, turkey breast or lean wild game to reduce your levels of bad eicosanoids like the Ugandans.

Chapter Twenty One

Refined Bread

Why spend money on what is not bread, and your labor on what does not satisfy? Listen, listen to me, and eat what is good and your soul will delight in the richest of fare. (Isaiah 55:2, Good News Bible, Good News Translation).

Let's first acknowledge that by definition, to refine means to separate and remove the purities from a food. Having stated that, you know where I am going with this chapter. Let's start by taking a closer look at how we get white flour from wheat. Wheat is the world's leading cereal and was cultivated first by African people. It provides us with all the necessary nutritional and vital elements that the body needs to function. It is used to make breads, pasta, cakes, cereals and many other healthy foods, but is processed to an unhealthy state. Ask yourself, why is most bread and flour white when the wheat it comes from is not? Common sayings in nutrition are, "if it starts off white, it just ain't right," "if your bread is brown, you'll stay around," "the whiter the bread, the sooner you're dead" and "colored foods gives good moods." These sayings are right on point and should be remembered when making food selections and passed on to our children.

The process of refining whole grain wheat into white flour, in my opinion, is an abomination to God since it consists of the dismantling of a pleasantly wholesome, perfectly constructed, life-giving, energy-yielding plant. Refining separates and removes at least 80% of the nutrients from the whole grain of wheat and then bleaches it white to make it more appealing to the eye. A wheat kernel's major parts include the bran, the germ and the endosperm. The bran is located at the outermost part of the plant and is about 15% of the grain. It is rich in vitamins, many minerals and fiber. The wheat germ is the next layer anatomically and it has a nourishing supply of the B and E vitamins and is about 5% of the grain. The innermost part of the plant is the endosperm which is about 85% of the grain.

A grain of wheat houses most of its nutritious elements at its outer layers. It is the outer aspect of the grain that is refined or removed during this process. There goes your vitamin A, E, B6, B12 and C, niacin, riboflavin, thiamine, inositol, folic acid, folinic acid, biotin, calcium, phosphorus, magnesium, sodium, potassium, iron, copper, manganese, zinc and other vital substances. Refiners attempt to replace many of the vitamins, thiamin, niacin, riboflavin and iron, but the nutritious value remains under par. Be sure to pay close attention before grabbing your favorite brand of bread off the grocery store shelf. Manufacturers use misleading wording to make these highly refined breads appear to be healthy. You can easily identify these breads as they are referred to as being "enriched."

Chapter Twenty Two

Nutrigenetics

"Jacob, however, took fresh-cut branches from poplar, almond and plane trees (chestnut) and made white stripes on them by peeling the bark and exposing the white inner wood of the branches. Then he placed the peeled branches in all the watering troughs, so that they would be directly in front of the flocks when they came to drink. When the flocks were in heat and came to drink, they mated in front of the branches. And they bore young that were streaked or speckled or spotted. Jacob set apart the young of the flock by themselves, but made the rest face the streaked and dark-colored animals that belonged to Laban. Thus he made separate flocks for himself and did not put them with Laban's animals. Whenever the stronger females were in heat, Jacob would place the branches in the troughs in front of the animals so they would mate near the branches, but if the animals were weak, he would not place them there. So the weak animals went to Laban and the strong ones to Jacob. In this way the man grew exceedingly prosperous and came to own large flocks, and maidservants and menservants, and camels and donkeys." (Genesis 30:37-43, NIV).

In the above story of Jacob, Laban, his father-in-law, cheated him out of his pledged wife. Jacob had offered to work for Laban seven years to be married to Rachel. However, on the wedding night, Laban switched daughters and gave him Leah. In the light of the next day, Jacob discovered the switch, but Laban would not offer Jacob Rachel as his wife unless he agreed to work another seven years for him. After the second seven years were completed, Jacob asked to be allowed to leave, but Laban did not want him to leave, since Jacob had greatly increased Laban's flocks and herds. Laban offered Jacob to take some of his animals, so Jacob chose the black, spotted, and striped ones for himself. Jacob separated the spotted and striped animals and kept them separated from Laban's flocks. During Bible study, many of us are taught that in this story Jacob believed that by putting striped rods in front of where the animals mated that more striped and spotted animals would be born. Is that what Jacob was thinking? Could it be that Jacob added the tree's nutrients to the water, the animals drank the water and the nutrients influenced their genes?

Well, this is what scientists are doing today!

The day is coming when, during your annual physical examination, your primary health care provider will take an extra vial of blood for a test to determine what foods you should and should not be eating. A computerized meter will analyze your DNA and recommend a diet to keep your body disease free and in tip top shape. The premise is simple: diet is a major factor in chronic disease and is responsible, research shows, for most types of cancer. Dietary chemicals (food) change the expression of your genes and even the genome itself. The influence of diet on health depends on an individual's genetic makeup. Nutritional geneticists realize that food not only is metabolized to provide your body energy, it also binds to proteins involved in "turning on" and "turning off" certain genes. A diet that's particularly out of balance, nutritional-genomics scientists say, will cause gene expressions that

189

nudge us toward diseases unless a precisely-tailored "intelligent diet" is employed to restore the equilibrium.

The genome of an organism is its whole hereditary information and is encoded in the DNA. This includes the genes and the non-coding sequences of the DNA. Genes carry information for making all the proteins required by all organisms. These proteins determine, among other things, how the organism looks, how well its body metabolizes food or fights infection, and sometimes, even how it behaves. Nutrigenetics is the study and understanding of how food affects one's genes and the science of matching a person's nutritional requirements to his or her genes. Until recently, it wasn't possible to know what weak links might be hidden in our genes. By testing an individual's DNA for common single mutations, it has become possible to formulate specific recommendations for diet changes. Our genes undergo these mutations when their DNA sequence changes. These changes can take place after interacting with the environment. The result is disease.

The most familiar example is explained in my earlier discussion on milk. If you're of northern European ancestry, you can probably digest milk, but if you're of African descent, you probably can't. In most mammals the gene for lactose tolerance switches off once an animal is weaned off of the mother's breast milk. All humans shared that fate until a mutation in the DNA of an isolated population of northern Europeans around 10,000 years ago introduced an adaptive post-wean tolerance to milk. The likelihood that you are intolerant to milk depends on the degree to which you have genes closet to the original man.

Geneticists agree that ALL of mankind (every single person alive today) is a descendent of a population of anatomically modern humans that existed in Africa until about 100,000 years ago. It was this group of people, nomads, who were responsible for populating the rest of the globe. This migration out of Africa was the beginning of races as we know them today. As humans traveled, they continued to evolve, and as our bodies interacted with new foods, we were self-selected for these naturally occurring variants. And, certain populations have variants that, when presented with different and new food, cause their genes to mutate and produce disease.

Plenty of examples bear witness to the interactions between certain cultures and certain diets - suggesting, if not proving, some interplay of genes and nutrition: Japanese who relocated to the United States after the Second World War quickly saw their cholesterol levels convert from high to low. The Alaskan Inuit, had high metabolisms that matched their activity levels. They would spend hours looking for high-fat food and had high metabolisms to make this hard work possible. They were saddled with an evolutionary disadvantage when they began living in heated homes and riding on snowmobiles instead of walking many miles per day. They now suffer from high levels of obesity, diabetes and cardiovascular disease. The Masai of East Africa have developed new health problems since exchanging their wild meat and blood diet for corn and beans.

Nutrigenetics is still a very young science. According to Infoholix Health News, its roots are tied to Prime Minister Tony Blair and President Bill Clinton's Human Genome Project from 1990.[1] If used properly, nutrigenetics can promote healthier and longer lives by guiding our choices on foods based on our genetic make-up.

Chapter Twenty Three

Vitamins and Minerals

"But the true servants of God shall be well provided for, feasting on fruit and honored in the gardens of delight..." (Koran 37:40-48).

A Chemist, in the early 1900's, by the name of Casimir Funk noticed that white rice (an unnatural processed food) was void of a substance that he used to cure a paralyzed pigeon. The pigeon suffered from a disease now known as berberi. He introduced Europe to idea that certain substances in foods can be used to cure diseases. A fact Africans had already known for millions of years. This mystery nutrient contained nitrogen and was a part of a group of chemicals called *amines*. Since it prolonged life, he named this and other similar substances *vitamines*. This tag was appropriate since the word *vita* means life and these chemicals are vital to all living organisms. This particular mystery substance, that cured beriberi, was eventually discovered and called thi*amine*. As time went on, more life saving chemicals were discovered that did not contain nitrogen, and were therefore not in the amine group. Hence, scientists took off the "e" and just called them vitamins. Thiamine is also known as vitamin B1.

Vitamins are essential organic (from plants or animals) nutrients found in the food you eat. They are needed in small amounts for maintaining health, normal growth and for physical activity. With only a few exceptions, the body cannot manufacture or synthesize vitamins. Vitamins are made within the leaves of plants. Animals have to eat plants to have access to most vitamins. And, man has to eat the plants (and/or animals) to have access to the vitamins. They also help regulate your metabolism, help convert your foods (protein, fat and carbohydrates) into energy, and are vital in the production of strong bones and tissue. Many of my patients think that taking vitamin supplements (instead of eating a proper balanced diet) is a safe thing to do. The fact of the matter is that vitamins cannot be converted into substances suitable for their incorporation into your tissues without food being present. This is why they should be taken with or shortly after eating.

All vitamins have a chemical name and a designated letter. For example, vitamin C is also known as ascorbic acid. There are at least nine vitamins in the vitamin B family: thiamin (B1), riboflavin (B2), niacin (B3), pantothenic acid (B5), pyridoxine (B6), folic acid, cobalamin (B12), inosital and biotin. Other vitamins are A, D, E and K. Vitamin K was so named after Coagulation, which means to clot, since vitamin K was found to help with clotting.

Vitamins are classified into two groups depending upon whether or not they dissolve in fat or in water. Fat-soluble vitamins (vitamins A, D, E and K) dissolve in fat to carry out their bodily functions. Any excess of these vitamins are stored in your liver. As you are probably thinking, people with liver disease may have a problem with storing these types of vitamins. Since they can be stored, they are not needed every day in your diet. In contrast, water-soluble vitamins dissolve in water and are not stored and any extra are eliminated in your urine. You must provide yourself with a continuous supply of them in your food. The water-soluble vitamins are the vitamin Bs (the B-complex group) and vitamin C. Water-soluble vitamins are easily destroyed or washed out of your foods during food storage or preparation. Learning proper storage and preparation of food can minimize vitamin loss. To do this, always:

1. Drink the water in which the food was cooked.
2. Keep your grains away from strong light.
3. Keep your fresh produce refrigerated at all times.
4. Store your milk in a non-transparent container.
5. Always ask God to bless your food with the proper nutrients needed for a healthy body.

Minerals are living proof that God intended for man and the universe to be on one accord. A mineral is a substance that occurs naturally in non-living things. They are commonly found in metals, water and rocks yet are needed by all living things. Plants need minerals and they get them from the water and soil. Animals (including humans) get them from the water and by eating plants.

Minerals are divided into two classifications: major mineral and trace elements. Major minerals are essential for human beings and are:

1) Sodium
2) Potassium
3) Chloride
4) Calcium
5) Magnesium
6) Phosphorus
7) Sulfur

Trace elements are also minerals but are present in animals in a very small amount in comparison to major minerals. They include:

1) Iron
2) Copper
3) Sclenium
4) Zinc
5) Iodine
6) Fluoride
7) Chromium
8) Manganese
9) Molybdenum

Essential Vitamins

Vitamin A (Retinol)

Vitamin A is the moisturizing nutrient. It keeps mucous membranes (eyes, nose, mouth, throat, vagina, and rectum) smooth and supple. It also boosts the immune system and enhances eye sight.

Fat-soluble; no daily consumption required.

Need: Eye, skin and adequate function of the immune system. It also helps maintain hair, bones and teeth.

Deficiency: dry eyes and night blindness, decreased hair growth, loss of appetite, dry skin a decreased immune system.

Overdose: Headache, bone pain, blurred vision, fatigue, diarrhea, irregular periods, joint pain, hair loss, dry and cracked skin.

Source: Carrots, squash, broccoli, green leafy vegetables, liver, fortified (added to) milk, other fortified foods and drinks.

Vitamin A Precursor, Pro-vitamin A (Beta Carotene)

Vitamin A Precursor, Pro-vitamin A (Beta Carotene) is the moisturizing nutrient. It keeps mucous membranes (eyes, nose, mouth, throat, vagina, and rectum) smooth and supple. It also boosts the immune system and enhances eye sight.

Fat-soluble; no daily consumption required.

Need: converts to vitamin A by the liver. Possesses anti-cancer properties as an antioxidant.

Deficiency: xerophthalmia (dry eyes), blindness. Weakened immune system.

Overdose: see vitamin A.

Source: Carrots, squash, green vegetables, broccoli.

Vitamin B1 (Thiamin)

Thiamin is a substance that works in conjunction with enzymes (a coenzyme). It is used in processes in which the body gets energy from carbohydrates. It also is a diuretic.

Water-Soluble; daily consumption required.

Need: Propagation of nerve function, muscle coordination and carbohydrate metabolism.

Deficiency: muscle cramps, anxiety, hysteria, depression, loss of appetite and paralysis (in extreme cases; beriberi).

Overdose: Unknown. An excess of any of the B vitamins may cause a deficiency of the others.

Source: Whole and enriched (added to) grains, Pork, sunflower seeds and dried beans.

Vitamin B2 (Riboflavin)

Like thiamin, riboflavin is also a coenzyme. It is essential for the breakdown of carbohydrates and proteins. And like vitamin A, it helps mucous membranes.

Water-soluble; daily consumption required.

Need: Needed for the metabolism of proteins, sugars and fats, essential to the function of vitamin B6 and vitamin B3, increases energy produced by food.

Deficiency: visual problems, dry cracking skin usually at the corner of the mouth and nose, sore tongue and mouth, anemia.

Overdose: unknown. An excess of can cause a deficiency of any of the other vitamins.

Source: Spinach, Milk, Liver, Mushrooms, enriched food (e.g. bread, noodles).

Vitamin B3 (Niacin)

Niacin is one name for a pair (nicotinic acids and nicotinamide) of naturally occurring nutrients. It is essential for proper growth and enzyme reactions. And like Thiamin, it helps with appetite and the breakdown of sugars and fats.

Water-soluble; daily consumption required.

Need: Improves circulation, decreases blood cholesterol, metabolizes proteins, sugars and fats, healthy digestive tract and nervous system, increases energy produced by foods, maintains healthy hair, skin, nails and tongue, and prevents pellagra (disease characterized by skin changes, diarrhea, nerve dysfunction and mental disturbances).

Deficiency: Pellagra (dry skin, nerve dysfunction, mental deterioration and diarrhea), gastrointestinal problems, nervousness, headaches, mouth sores, insomnia, dermatitis, bad breath and mental depression.

Overdose: niacin flush (dermatitis, hot flashes), high blood sugars and increased uric acid production, abnormal heart beats and liver disease.

Source: Tuna, Chicken, Beef, Peanuts, Mushrooms, Bran and enriched grains.

Vitamin B5 (Pantothenic Acid)

Pantothenic acid is needed for hormone production and carbohydrate breakdown. It also helps stabilize blood sugar levels, fight infections and protects red blood cells.

Water-soluble; daily consumption required.

Need: needed for the utilization of vitamins, improves body's resistance to stress, maturation for the nervous system, needed to make adrenal hormones and chemicals that regulate nerve function and to release energy from carbohydrates, fats and proteins.

Deficiency: growth retardation, dizzy spells, digestive problems, painful and burning feet and muscle cramps.

Overdose: may lead to a deficiency of other B vitamins.

Source: animal tissues, legumes and whole grain cereals.

Vitamin B6 (Pyridoxine)
Pyridoxine is a component of enzymes that metabolize fats and proteins and removes an excessive amount of homocysteine (a dangerous amino acid released with protein breakdown).

Water-soluble; daily consumption required.

Need: build-up and breakdown of protein, carbohydrates and fat, healthy skin, proper balance of sodium and phosphorus, red blood cell formation, promotes nerve and brain function. It decreases homocysteine levels.

Deficiency: Prevents toxic buildup of homocysteine, anemia, nervousness, irritability, itchy and scaling skin, insomnia, slow learning and loss of hair. High levels of homocysteine lead to increased risks of heart disease.

Overdose: Nerve damage.

Source: Animal protein, spinach, bananas and broccoli.

Vitamin B9 (Folic acid)

An essential nutrient for humans that is needed in the production of DNA, the breakdown of protein, and the subsequent synthesis of amino acids used to produce new body tissues.

Water-soluble; daily consumption required.

Need: manufacturing of genetic material (DNA and RNA), amino acid metabolism, red blood cell formation and reduces the risk of neural tube defects in newborns. It lowers homocysteine levels.

Deficiency: Prevents toxic buildup of homocysteine, anemia, gastrointestinal problems, Vitamin B12 deficiency, diarrhea and pre-mature gray hair. Deficiency produces an increased risk of heart disease and colon cancer.

Overdose: Seizures.

Source: Green vegetables, orange juice, organ meat, sprouts.

Vitamin B12 (Cobalamin)

Cobalamin is responsible for making healthy red blood cells, protecting nerves and allowing nerve endings to communicate.

Water-soluble; daily consumption required.

Need: Prevents toxic buildup of homocysteine, energy, formation and regeneration of red blood cells, metabolism of carbohydrates, proteins & fat, healthy nervous system, promotes growth in children and calcium absorption.
Deficiency (rare except in strict vegetarians and elderly with inability to absorb): Anemia (pernicious), nerve damage, growth retardation in children, fatigue, depression, lack of balance and brain damage. A deficiency lowers homocysteine levels.

<u>Overdose</u>: may lead to a deficiency of other B vitamins. An overdose increased risk of heart disease.

<u>Source</u>: Animal meat only.

Vitamin H (Biotin)

Biotin is known as hair, skin and nails nutrient as it is in abundance in over-the-counter supplements that claim to be healthy for those parts of the body. It does so by providing cells with fatty acids and amino acids after metabolism.

<u>Water-soluble</u>; daily consumption required.

<u>Need</u>: healthy hair, skin and nails, aids in utilization of protein, vitamin B9 (folic acid), vitamin B5 (pantothenic acid) & vitamin B12 (cobalamin) and sugar metabolism.

<u>Deficiency</u>: extreme exhaustion, seborrhic dermatitis in infants, drowsiness, loss of appetite, grayish skin color.

Source: Cheese, eggs, yolk, peanut butter and cauliflower.

Inositol

Inositol is found in plant and animal tissue and classified as a member of the vitamin B complex.

It is part of a phospholipid found in the brain of humans.

Water-soluble; daily consumption required.

Need: proper formation of cell membranes. Improves nerve transmission, helps in breakdown & transporting fats within the body, necessary for the formation of lecithin, helps prevent hair thinning and helps lower cholesterol levels, brain cell nutrition, prevents atherosclerosis and has anti-cancer properties. Deficiency: elevated cholesterol levels, hair loss, constipation, eczema.

Overdose: decreased calcium, iron and zinc absorption, uterine contractions in pregnancy.

Source: oranges, nuts, beans, wheat, wheat bran, cantaloupe, blackstrap molasses, brewer's yeast, grapefruit, meat.

PABA (Para-amino benzoic Acid)

Water-soluble; daily consumption required.

Need: Red blood cell production, enhances the effects of cortisone, increases fertility in women, protein metabolism, prevents gray hair & returns hair to its natural color, intestinal bacterial activity, removes free radicals and production of vitamin B9 (folic acid).

Deficiency: eczema, fatigue, irritability, depressions, nervousness, constipation, headaches, digestive disorders, gray hair,

Overdose: Low blood sugars, rash, fever and liver damage.

Source: Wheat germ, animal food, grains, eggs, beef liver, blackstrap molasses, brewer's yeast.

Vitamin C (Ascorbic acid)

An antioxidant that boosts the immune system, reduces the severity of allergic reactions, aids in hormone production and wound healing and in high levels slows the development of cataracts.

Fat-soluble; no daily consumption required.

Need: One of the body's most power antioxidants (see free radicals and antioxidants). It yields healthy teeth, bones & gums. Collagen formation for healing wounds, scars & bones, prevention and treatment of colds, red blood cell viability, some anti-cancer effects by blocking nitrate conversion when tobacco smoke, bacon, lunch meat and some vegetables are consumed, blood vessel strength and iron absorption. Helps lower cholesterol, reduces the risk of heart disease and cancer, boosts the immune system, and helps ward off infections and colds.

Deficiency: muscle weakness, bleeding gums, easy bruising and scurvy in extreme cases.

Overdose: unknown.

Source: oranges, red pepper, guava, grapefruit, papaya, strawberries, kiwi, tomatoes, parsley, green peppers and cauliflower.

Vitamin D

Vitamin D is referred to as the sunshine vitamin. It is actually a hormone but is considered a vitamin only because of the body's ability to manufacture it is dependent on environmental factors. It is the key to calcium and phosphorus utilization because without it your body cannot absorb and use them. Because of this, it is essential for strong bones and teeth. Evidence now suggests that without it increases your chance of getting diabetes and some forms of cancer. It comes in three forms: calciferol, cholecalciferol, and ergocalciferol. Calciferol occurs naturally in egg yolk and fish oil. It is added to (fortified) milk and margarine. Cholecalciferol is the substance produced when sunlight interacts with the melanin in your skin. Ergocalciferol is the substance made when sunlight interacts with the color pigment in plants. Cholecalciferol raises blood levels more effectively than the others.

Fat-soluble; no daily consumption required.

Need: Calcium absorption in the intestines; bone formation phosphorus metabolism, skin respiration, helps build and maintain teeth, blood clotting, nervous system function, anti-bone tumor action, inhibits intestinal tumors.

Deficiency: soft bones; osteoporosis, Rickets in children.
Overdose: Calcification of organs, bone fragility, cardiovascular disease, kidney damage.

Source: Skin exposure to the sun (see Melanin), Egg, Eel, Milk, fish (sardines, halibut, salmon, tuna, herring), beef liver.

Vitamin E

Vitamin E is an antioxidant that is need by all animals, including you. It is needed to maintain a healthy reproductive system.

Fat-soluble; no daily consumption required.

Need: Antioxidant and free radical scavenger (see Free Radicals and Antioxidants), slows the aging process, red blood cell formation, preserves fatty acids, fertility, nervous system function, body tissues production, muscle fiber and blood vessel production, protects fat soluble vitamins, pituitary gland protection, iron absorption, adrenal and sex hormones, cell respiration and anti-cancer.

Deficiency: Rare. Can causes nervous system abnormalities. Deficiencies are usually seen in premature or low birth weight babies with fat absorption abnormalities.

Overdose: Unknown.

Source: All seeds, nuts, beans, corn & peas, corn and cotton seed oil, butter, brown rice, wheat germ and soybean oils, eggs, oatmeal, beef liver, human milk, alfalfa, lettuce and tomatoes.

Vitamin K

Vitamin K is composed of a group of chemicals that your body uses to make substances that are needed for blood clotting. It is also needed to make bone and kidney tissues.

Fat-soluble; no daily consumption required.

Need: Helps blood to clot, prevents bleeding, prevents bruising, prevents osteoporosis, can be manufactured by acidophilus (*Lactobacillus acidophilus* is the most commonly "friendly" bacteria), and destroyed by antibiotics.

Source: green leafy vegetables, made in intestines, liver, eggs, yogurt, alfalfa, tomatoes, oatmeal, fish soy oil and yogurt.

Calcium

Calcium is about 2-3 pounds of your total body weight. It is packed within your bones and teeth. On the cellular level, it makes it possible for cells to send messages to one another. It also regulates your blood pressure and movement of your muscles.

Need: strong bones and teeth, nervous and musculoskeletal systems, activate enzymes for food metabolism and blood clotting.

Deficiency: Soft brittle bones; Rickets in children.

Overdose: Constipation, kidney stones, build-up in tissues and blocks absorption of other minerals (e.g. iron).

Source: Yogurt, milk, cheese, sardines, greens, turnips and broccoli.

Potassium

Need: nerve communication, muscle function and helps maintains fluid balance.

Deficiency: muscle weakness, paralysis, muscle cramps, irritability, and anorexia.

Overdose: cardiac malfunction, death.

Source: Bananas, peanuts, orange juice, green beans, sunflower seeds, broccoli and mushrooms.

Iron

Need: essential for the production of the hemoglobin found inside of red blood cells. They are responsible for transporting oxygen of body tissues.

Deficiency: anemia, shortness of breath, weakness, numbness and tingling, skin pallor, headaches, fainting.

Overdose: Toxicity to the liver and heart.

Source: animal liver, lean meats, kidney beans, enriched foods, and raisins. Spinach (oxalic acid) and some grains and legumes inhibit iron absorption.

Phosphorus

Need: serves in production of bones (with calcium) and teeth, nerve and muscle function as well as metabolism.

Deficiency: Anorexia, weakness & bone weakness and pain.

Overdose: prevents calcium absorption.

Source: chicken breasts, eggs, nuts, some legumes and dairy products.

Magnesium

Need: production of genetic materials, enzyme production, and bone growth.

Deficiency: energy production, gene production and bone growth.

Overdose: nausea, vomiting & diarrhea, neuropathies and low blood pressure.

Source: spinach, beef, cashews, bran, broccoli, tofu and popcorn.

Chapter Twenty Four

Glycemic Index

The Glycemic Index (GI) is a numerical value assigned to carbohydrates (long chain sugars). This ranking, initially created for diabetics, should be used by everyone in order to control hunger, stabilize blood sugar levels and prevent insulin resistance and diabetes. The GI of a particular food is usually based on how fast the particular food is broken down and thus increases your blood sugar levels. The GI is compared to sugar (glucose) since it is thought to have the highest GI out of the foods we commonly eat. Therefore glucose is given the value of 100.

Foods with high GI indices will raise blood sugar levels rapidly. On the other hand, foods with low GI scores will release their sugars into the blood at a slower rate. The lower the GI is for a particular food, the healthier it is (because, the slower it is broken down and the slower your blood sugar increases) It is therefore important that you have an idea of the Glycemic Index values of the variety of foods you consume.

The act of eating should be looked upon as a behavior necessary to maintain life and not as an act of pleasure. The food you eat should be chosen meticulously, out of self-respect and with a great deal of knowledge. You were given taste buds so that you would get a sense of enjoyment out of eating, differentiate between different foods and to entice you to continue to eat. However, it is easy to become consumed with the taste of food and this gluttony leads to poor choices, unhealthiness and a shortened life span. The illnesses that result from food obsession are often preceded by undesirable symptoms such as postprandial fatigue, weakness, lightheadedness, episodes of low blood sugars, weight gain and depression. Often times, this is a result of the excessive consumption of carbohydrates with a high GI over a long period of time.

How one is affected by high GI foods depends upon factors that influence the digestion and absorption rate of the particular food. Some of the factors are:

the age of the food (i.e. ripeness), the serving size, the degree of processing, the manner of preparation, the time of the day consumed, your health status and your metabolism.

Foods with high Glycemic Indices stimulate the pancreas to produce high levels of insulin. This rise in blood insulin levels quickly lower the blood sugar levels as the sugar is moved into the cells for energy. As the blood sugar drops, there is a subsequent drop in blood insulin levels as well. It is this rapid drop in insulin that starts the formation of fat. Once insulin levels are equal to or below the GI threshold, your brain responds by igniting the hunger cascade. Eating more high GI foods begets more hunger, overweight and obesity. You are then introduced to early or unnecessary coronary artery disease, strokes, kidney failure and cancers, to name a few.

The Glycemic Index of Common Foods

Low Glycemic index foods = less than 55.

Medium Glycemic index foods = 55-70.

High Glycemic index foods = more than 70.

Low Glycemic Foods

Bakery Products: pound cake (54)

Fruit: bananas (54), kiwi, grapes (46), oranges (44), peaches (42), plums (39), pears (38), apples (38), dried apricots (31), grapefruit (25), cherries (22).

Beverages: soy milk (30), apple juice (41), carrot juice (45), pineapple juice (46), grapefruit juice (48), orange juice (52).

Breads: multi-grain (48), whole grain (50).

Breakfast Cereals: All-Bran (42), non-instant oatmeal (49).

Cereal grains: barley (25), rye (34), wheat kernels (41), instant rice (46), parboiled rice (48), cracked barley (50).

Dairy Foods: low-fat ice-cream (50), 2% milk (34), skimmed milk (32), fat-free milk (32), whole milk (27), chocolate milk (24), low-fat yogurt (14).

Pasta: macaroni (45), white spaghetti (41), meat filled ravioli (39), whole wheat spaghetti (37), protein enriched spaghetti (27), vermicelli (35), fettuccine (32).

Root Crop: sweet potato (54), yams (51), cooked carrots (39).

Sweets and Snack Foods: M&Ms (peanuts) (32), snickers (40), chocolate bar 30g (49), jams and marmalades (49).

Soups: canned tomato soup (38), canned lentil soup (44).

Vegetables and beans: artichoke (15), asparagus (15), broccoli (15), cauliflower (15), celery (15), cucumber (15), eggplant (15), peanuts (15), green beans (15), lettuce (all) (15), low-fat yogurt with artificial sweetener (15), pepper (all) (15), snow peas (15), spinach (15), young summer squash (15), tomatoes (15), zucchini (15), boiled soy beans (16), dried peas (22), boiled lentils (29), chickpeas (33), boiled haricot (38), black-eyed beans (41), canned chickpeas (42), canned baked beans (48), canned kidney beans (52), canned lentils (52).

Medium Glycemic Foods

Bakery Products: danish pastry (59), unsweetened muffin (62), tart cake (65), angel cake (67), croissant (67).

Biscuits: sweetmeal/cornmeal biscuits (58), shortbread (64), water biscuits (65).

Breads: pita bread, white (57), cheese pizza (60), hamburger bun (61), rye-flour bread (64), whole grain bread (69).

Breakfast Cereals: oat bran (55), muesli (56), mini wheats, whole grain (57), shredded wheat (69).

Cereal grains: brown rice (55), wild rice (57), white rice (58), barley flakes (66), taco shell (68).

Dairy Foods: Ice-cream (61), fruit cocktail (55), mangoes (56), apricots (57), apricots canned in syrup (64), raisins (64), pineapple (66).

Pasta: durum wheat spaghetti (55), macaroni cheese (64).

Root Crop: boiled potato (56), new potato (57), canned potato (61), beetroot (61), steamed potato (65), mashed potato (70).

Sweets and Snack Foods: popcorn (55), mars bar (64), table sugar (sucrose) (65).

Soups: Canned black bean (64), canned green pea (66).

High Glycemic Foods

Bakery Products: waffles (76), doughnuts (76).

Biscuits: water biscuits (65), rice cakes (77).

Breads: white bread (71), white rolls (73), baguette (95).

Breakfast Cereals: golden grahams (71), puffed wheat (74), weetabix (77), rice krispies (82), cornflakes (83).

Cereal Grains: millet (71).

Fruits: watermelon (72).

Pasta: brown rice pasta (92).

Root Crop: chips (75), micro waved potato (82), instant potato (83), baked potato (85), and parsnips (97).

Sweets and Snack Foods: corn chips (74), jelly beans (80), pretzels (81), dates (103).

Vegetables and Beans: broad beans (79).

In short, low GI foods are slower to digest, so you feel satiated (full) longer. This is exactly what you need to lose weight, eat less and live longer. Keeping your blood insulin levels low inhibits the formation of fat and assists in the conversion of fat back into energy. This is how low GI foods help you lose weight. Choosing low glycemic foods more often than not is a sure way to maintain your ideal body weight forever.

Chapter Twenty Five

Sleep

"The sleep of a laboring man is sweet, whether he eats little or much..." (Ecclesiastes 5:12. Holy Bible, King James Version).

There is a direct correlation between how much sleep one gets and one's total body weight. Sleep can be considered a state of decreased consciousness and physical activity which normally occurs at night. It is the time when man (and other animals) slows down so that that their bodies can undergo repairs. Sleep is necessary for the maintenance and rejuvenation of mental and physical health. The sleep cycle involves distinct phases that alternate cyclically from light sleep to deep, then deeper and deepest sleep throughout the sleep period.

At least 1/3 of our life in spent sleeping. One-third of 24 hours is 8 hours, hence the recommendation that the "ideal" amount of daily sleep is 8 hours. According to a University of Chicago

Chronicle article, entitled *Lack of sleep alters hormones and metabolism*, the average night's sleep decreased from about nine hours in 1910 to about 7.5 hours in 1975.[1] If this truly reflects a downward trend as they claim, what do you think the average night's sleep was 6 billion years ago?

Scientists found that depriving rats of sleep led to their early demise. In fact, without any sleep, they didn't live for longer than a few weeks. They lost their ability to maintain cognitive (thought) processes, body temperature and a normal immune system. They eventually became overwhelmed with infection and died.

According to National Sleep Foundation's (NSF) CEO, Richard L. Gelula, "Obesity has become an epidemic in this country, and so has sleep deprivation. We now believe that these two are linked more closely than we thought."[2] And, the National Sleep Foundation's 2002 *Sleep in America* poll found that a significant number of adults (39%) get less than the recommended 7-9 hours of sleep on weeknights, and nearly one-quarter reported they were more likely to eat more when they didn't get enough sleep.[3]

It has been found that when you don't get enough sleep, your body has too little leptin and too much ghrelin. Yes, this link between sleep and obesity seems all to be related to a hormone called *leptin* and a hormone called *ghrelin*. Leptin is a hormone produced by fat cells (adipocytes) that regulates the amount of food you want to eat and the amount of energy burned within your body. In other words, Leptin interacts with your brain, specifically at the hypothalamus and the thyroid gland, and tells it that you have had enough food, get rid the sensation of hunger and burn away some of the fat you hate so much. When your body needs to make energy, it converts your stored fat into energy. It is the ideal chemical for metabolism boosting and weight loss. During sleep, leptin levels increase, telling your brain you have plenty of energy for the time being and there's no need to trigger the feeling of hunger or the burning of calories. When you don't get your eight hours of sleep, you end up with too little leptin in your body, which, through a series of steps, makes your brain think you don't have enough energy for your needs. So your brain tells you that you are hungry, even though you don't actually need food at that time. Your body then goes in the starvation mode and you began to store (as fat) everything you eat. The decrease in leptin brought on by sleep deprivation can result in a constant feeling of hunger and a general slow-down of your metabolism and hence weight gain, overweight then obesity. Is lack of sleep making you fat?

Ghrelin, on the other hand, is produced by the stomach and increases hunger and fat storage in the body. It actually does the exact opposite of leptin. In the state of sleep deprivation, your stomach produces excess ghrelin. It tells the brain that it is hungry, to stop breaking down your stored fat and make as much fat as it can. With adequate sleep, ghrelin levels decrease and your metabolic functions increase, therefore you burn fat and aren't hungry.

Why does this sleep-hunger correlation even exist? When your ancestors began to mobilize out of Africa in search of animal herds, more fertile soil and decent climates, the winter months meant shorter days, longer nights and less food. Man therefore needed to develop an evolutionary process to allow him to burn fewer calories since he spent more hours sleeping. With the grace of God, we began to produce leptin and ghrelin. This allowed us to keep our weight and hunger in check. Today, we are not the resting (sleeping) humans that our bodies have evolved into, and expect us to be. The lack of sleep could be contributing our community's epidemic of obesity.

Resting has got to be godly as even God rested: *"And on the seventh day God ended his work which he had made; and he rested on the seventh from all his work which he had made."* (Genesis 2:2, Holy Bible, King James Version).

Chapter Twenty Six

The Plant: God's Medicine

"And by the river upon the bank thereof, on this side and on that side, shall grow all trees for meat, whose leaf shall not fade, neither shall the fruit thereof be consumed: it shall bring forth new fruit according to his months, because their waters they issued out the sanctuary: and the fruit thereof shall be for meat, and the leaf thereof for medicine." (Ezekiel 47:12. Holy Bible, Original African Heritage Edition).

Herbal medicine is the oldest form of healthcare known to all of mankind. Herbs had been used by all cultures throughout the history of man. It is estimated that over 4 billion people, 80 percent of the world's population, use a form of herbal medicine for some aspect of their primary health care. An herb is a plant whose stem is not woody or persistent. In some cultures, herbs are used to treat a variety of disorders ranging from the common cold to sexually transmitted diseases and diabetes.

The oldest known written records detailing the use of herbs in the treatment of illnesses are the Mesopotamian clay tablet writings and the Egyptian papyrus. Africans have been using herbal medicines well before they began recording these God given practices. It was about 4000 B.C. when King Assurbanipal of Sumeria ordered the compilation of the first known *materia medica*; an ancient form of today's United States Pharmacopoeia (a government published book containing descriptions of drugs). It contained some 250 herbal drugs (including garlic, still a favorite of herbal doctors). The Ebers Papyrus, the most important of the preserved Egyptian manuscripts, was written around 1500 B.C. and includes even earlier herbal information. It contains 876 prescriptions made up of more than 500 different substances, including many herbs. The medicinal parts put forward in this and other African texts formed the intellectual foundation of classical medical practice in Rome, Greece and the Arabic world.

Ailment	Herbal Treatment
Aching joints/Arthritis	*comfrey, celery, St John's Wort, borage, chamomile, gotu kola*
Aching muscles	*ginger, chamomile, marjoram, rose-scented geranium*
Acidity	*chamomile, fennel, mint*
Acne	*buchu, calendula, chamomile, cloves, comfrey, parsley, rosella*
AIDS/HIV	*echinacea, garlic, golden seal*
Alcoholism	*alfalfa, Melissa, milk thistle*
Allergies	*Echinacea*

Alzheimer's disease	**Rosemary**
Analgesic	**buchu, clover, cloves, lavender**
Anorexia	**Cardamom**
Anti-aging	**Borage, celery, lemon thyme, alfalfa, pennywort**
Antibacterial/Antibiotic	**Calendula, cinnamon, lavender, marjoram, turmeric, buchu, echinacea, alfalfa, rosemary,**
Anti-cancer	**Clover, lemon, gotu kola, turmeric**
Anticoagulant	**Turmeric, pennywort**
Antidepressant	**Sunlight exposure, jasmine, lavender, lemon verbena, Melissa, oat straw, rose hip, rosemary, St Johns wort**
Anti-inflammatory	**Omega-3 fish**

	oil, basil, bergamot, chamomile, clover, echinacea, ginger, lemon, rose hip, rosemary, yarrow
Anti-oxidant	Lemon, turmeric
Antiseptic	Bergamot, calendula, cloves, ginger, lavender, rose hip, yarrow
Anti-spasmodic	Anise, basil, cardamom, chamomile, cinnamon, cloves, lemon thyme, lemon verbena, marjoram, Melissa, rose hip, rosemary, St Johns wort, yarrow
Anti-viral	Echinacea, Melissa, rose hip, St Johns wort

Anxiety	Lavender, alfalfa, marjoram, mint, oat straw, rose-scented geranium
Asthma	Anise, cardamom, chamomile, cinnamon, echinacea, lemon thyme, maidenhair fern, stinging nettle, turmeric
Athletes foot	Buchu, calendula, marjoram, gotu kola
Baldness	Rosemary
Blood pressure (high)	Basil, celery, lemon, yarrow
Blood pressure (low)	Rosemary
Boils	Comfrey, echinacea, corn silk, golden seal, gotu kola
Breast cancer	Clover, violet
Bronchitis	Anise, cardamom, clover, comfrey,

	echinacea, elderflower, ginger, mullein, violet
Cholesterol (high)	Garlic, basil, celery, fennel, parsley, turmeric
Circulation (poor)	Ginger, gotu kola, rosemary, yarrow
Colds	Bergamot, echinacea, elderflower, ginger, lemon thyme, maidenhair fern, marjoram, pineapple sage, rose hip, rosella, sage, violet, yarrow, buchu, comfrey, alfalfa, mullein
Colic	Anise, caraway, cardamom, catmint, chamomile, fennel, lemon verbena, Melissa, mint,

	peppermint, rose hip, strawberry
Colitis	Calendula, Melissa, mint
Concentration (poor)	Gotu kola, peppermint, sage, Ginko
Bladder infecton	Borage, cardamom, goldenrod, corn silk
Diarrhea	Goldenrod, nutmeg, raspberry, rose hip, strawberrys
Digestive problems	Bergamot, Melissa, mint, oat straw, peppermint, strawberry
Diuretic	Borage, celery, fennel, lemon, corn silk, parsley, raspberry, rosemary, stinging nettle, strawberry, yarrow
Eczema	Borage, chamomile,

	clover, elderflower, stinging nettle, turmeric
Energy (to increase)	*Alfalfa, oat straw, peppermint, rosella, rosemary, chamomile, jasmine, lavender, rose-scented geranium*
Gas (Flatulence)	*Caraway, cardamom, catmint, lemon grass, marjoram, Melissa, mint, peppermint*
Flu	*Buchu, echinacea, ginger, lemon, Melissa, sage, yarrow*
Fungal infection	*Comfrey, echinacea, turmeric*
Gastric ulcers/ Gastroenteritis	*Calendula, Melissa, oat*

	straw
Gout	*Clover, fennel, parsley, stinging nettle, strawberry*
Hemorrhoids	*Catmint, gotu kola*
Hay fever	*Bergamot, chamomile, elderflower, stinging nettle, violet*
Headaches	*Catmint, ginger, violet*
Heartburn	*Anise, buchu, caraway, fennel, lemon grass, melissa, mint, nutmeg, peppermint, pineapple sage*
Impotence	*Anise, pennywort, tribulus terrestris, muira puama, yohimbine*
Indigestion	*Bergamot, catmint, chamomile, ginger, lemon*

	thyme
Irritable bowel syndrome	**Borage, oat straw**
Kidney stones	**Fennel, goldenrod, maidenhair fern, corn silk, rose hip**
Menopause	**Cinnamon, alfalfa, sage, St Johns wort,**
Menstruation (pain/cramps)	**Anise, parsley**
Multiple sclerosis	**oat straw**
Nausea	**Anise, bergamot, buchu, catmint, ginger, mint, nutmeg, turmeric**
Oily skin	**Basil, bergamot, alfalfa, oat straw**
Osteoporosis	**Comfrey, oat straw, parsley, sage**
Overactive thyroid	**Melissa**
Overeating	**Melissa, mint, peppermint**
Pain relief	**Chamomile,**

	cloves, oat straw, St Johns wort
Panic attacks	Lavender, melissa, oat straw, rose-scented, geranium
Prostate problems	Corn silk, raspberry, stinging nettle golden seal, pumpkin seeds, ginger
Psoriasis	Clover, parsley, turmeric
Skin cancer	Gotu kola
Thrush	Goldenrod
Toothache	Cloves
Vomiting	Bergamot, ginger, mint
Weight loss (help)	Celery, fennel, parsley

"Reading about nature is fine, but if a person walks in the woods and listens carefully, he can learn more than what is in books, for they speak with the voice of God," George Washington Carver.[1]

As the field of medicine began to develop in the United States, plants continued as a mainstay of medicine. The African-American culture maintained the use of plants by passing it as a family tradition. But, over time these treasures became lost. What did your grandmother do to combat her pregnancy related nausea and vomiting? Or, what did the "medicine man" give to the village people when he suspected a poisonous snake bite. The names of many herbs are familiar to many African-Americans but their healing properties are unknown. Several of the following commonly used herbs or their healing properties listed in the chart below may not sound familiar to many of us:

Commonly used names of healing herbs	How it Helps
Alfalfa, buffalo grass, Chilean clover	Prevent heart disease, lower cholesterol and help prevent strokes
Allspice, clove pepper, pimento, pimento, Jamaican pepper	Digestive aid, anesthetic, pain reliever and has been used to treat flatulence and diabetes
Aloe, socotrine, cape, curaiao, Barbados, Zanzibar aloe	Burns, scalds, scrapes, sunburn, anti-infection, skin beautifier
Anise, aniseed, sweet cumin	cough, digestive aid, menopause discomfort and prostate cancer
Lemon balm, bee balm, balm, sweet balm, melissa, cure-all	Wounds, herpes and other infections, digestive aid, tranquilizer
Basil, sweet basil, St Josephs wort	Infections, acne, immune system booster
Bay, sweet bay, green bay, laurel, Grecian or Roman laurel	Soothes sore joints, infections, excellent as additive to bathes for relaxation
Caraway, carum	Soothes digestive tract, helps expel gas, relief of menstrual cramps, uterine relaxation
Catnip, catnep, catsworth, catmint, field balm	Excellent for cold symptoms when used as a tea, sedative, tranquilizer, digestive aid, menstruation promoter, menstrual cramps,

240

	flatulence, colic
Chamomile, anthemis, matricaria, ground apple	*Considered a "cure-all,"*
Chicory, endive, chickory	*Reduces bitter taste of coffee's caffeine, cleanses urinary tract, digestive aid, mild laxative, gout and rheumatic disease*
Cinnamon, Ceylon cinnamon, Saigon cinnamon, cassia	*Infection prevention, pain relief, digestive aid, uterine relaxation*
Clove, clavos, caryophyllus	*Oil for toothache*
Coriander, cilantro, Chinese parsley	*Indigestion, flatulence, diarrhea, muscle and joint pains*
Cranberry	*Urinary tract infections (UTI), incontinence, vitamin C*
Dandelion, wild endive, lion's tooth, piss-in-bed	*Highly recommended for salads, add to bath for prevention of yeast infections, PMS, weight loss, high blood pressure, congestive heart failure, cancer prevention, yeast infections, digestive aids*
Dill	*add to bath to prevent UTI, infection prevention and fighter, soothing digestive aid, stomach aches, flatulence*
Echinacea, coneflower, purple coneflower	*Immune system booster, fights viral and bacteria infections, arthritis. **It is the most productive herb of all***

	times.
Eucalyptus, gum tree, blue gum, Australian Fever Tree	*Loosens phlegm, kills influenza, cure bronchitis, minor cuts, scrapes, repels cockroaches*
Fennel, finocchio, carosella, Florence Fennel	*Helps expel gas, colic, fights prostate cancer*
Feverfew, ferbrifuge plant, wild quinine, bachelor's button	*Excellent for migraine headaches, lower blood pressure and good for digestive aids*
Garlic, stinking rose, heal-all, poor man's treacle	*The world's oldest medicine, the world's wonder drug, wounds, cold symptoms, ringworm, high cholesterol, cardiovascular disease, high blood pressure, reduces blood clots, reduces blood sugar, eliminates lead and heavy metals in the bloodstream, help leprosy patients, fights cancers, helps AIDS patients, and many more*
Ginger, Asian ginger, African ginger, American ginger	*Motion and morning sickness, digestive aid, arthritis, cholesterol, blood pressure, heart attacks, blood clots*
Ginkgo, maidenhair tree	*The earth's oldest tree, increases blood flow to the brain, prevents strokes and heart attacks, improves memory and impotence, chronic dizziness, blindness,*

	circulation, asthma, tinnitus, deafness
Ginseng, root of immortality, man root, life root, seng seng	*Immune system booster, lowers cholesterol, lowers blood pressure, reduces heart attacks, protects the liver, helps increase appetites, helps cancer patients with radiation therapy. The root should be at least 6 years old.*
Horehound, marrubium, hoarhound, white horehound	*Respiratory symptoms and infections*
Hyssop	*Inhibits herpes simplex virus, cold symptoms*
Juniper, Geneva, genvrier	*A diuretic so it increases urine production, PMS, high blood pressure, congestive heart failure, arthritis*
Kelp, focus, seawrack, cutweed, bladderwrack, wakame, hijiki, kombu, arame	*Reduces heart disease, protects from heavy metals*
Lavender, English lavender	*Superb fragrance herb, makes a great bath addition,*
Marijuana, weed, herb, cannabis, pot, dope, sess	*Cancer, AIDS, glaucoma, appetitive enhancer in AIDS and cancer patients, nausea*
Marjoram, oregano, knotted marjoram	*Applied powdered herb rids herpes simplex 1 & 2, digestive aid*
Mint	*Wounds, burns, soothes stomach, morning sickness*
Mistletoe, Lignum	*Blood pressure, elevated heart*

cruces, herbe de la croix, viscum	rate, increases gastrointestinal mobility and uterine contractions
Myrrh, balsamodendron	Mouthwash, toothpaste
Nettle, stinging nettle, common nettle, greater nettle	Gout, hay fever, scurvy, PMS, heart disease
Red pepper, hot pepper, bell pepper	Flavoring foods during cooking, digestive aid, diarrhea, chronic pains, shingles, head aches
Rosemary, rosemarine, incensier	Preserver when added to wrapper meats, cooking, digestive aids, decongestant
Saffron, Spanish saffron	De-clogs arteries, lowers blood pressure, reduces cholesterol
Sage	Anti-perspirant, reduces blood sugar, sore throat, flavor in meats
Savory, white thyme, bean herb	Excellent culinary herb, expectorant, digestive aid
Skullcap, Quaker bonnet, mad dog weed, hoodwort, helmet flower	Tranquilizer, sedative, insomnia
Tarragon, dragon herb, estragon, French or Russian tarragon	Fresh leaves chewed for toothache, cuts, wounds, local anesthetic, prevents diseases
Tea, green tea, black tea, white tea	Calming effects, cold symptoms, asthma, diarrhea, tooth decay
Thyme, mother of	Fights bacterial and viral

thyme, common or garden thyme, wild, creeping or mother thyme	*infections, digestive aid, menstrual cramps, cough, emphysema, cuts wounds*
Valerian, phu, heal-all, garden valerian	*Tranquilizer (replacement for valium), reduces blood pressure*
Vervain, Indian hyssop, blue vervain, verbena	*Headache, arthritis, aspirin substitute, constipation*
Witch hazel, hamamelis, snapping hazelnut, winterbloom	*Astringent gargle, antiseptic, anesthetic, anti-inflammatory, cuts, bruises, hemorrhoids, sore muscles*
Yarrow, bloodwort, nose bleed, thousand weed, milfoil, soldier's woundwort	*Wounds, digestive aid, menstrual cramps, mild sedative*

Finally, America is taking a closer look at the herbs in Africa for their medicinal values. For example, a benefit of the pygeum (Pygeum africanum) plant is being considered as the treatment for urinary tract infections. Bridelia ferruginous (found in eastern and western grasslands) and Indigofera arrecta (found in tropical areas) are two African shrubs presently being investigated, and show promise, for the treatment of diabetes.

It is in my opinion that physicians have their hands tied when it comes to treating diseases. Medicine has defined "appropriate" treatments of particular diseases as "standard of care." As far as medications are concerned, the pharmaceutical industry defines which medications should be used for each disease. This is determined by the results of the research studies that they conduct. Not treating diseases the way pharmaceutical research suggests could result in a malpractice suit. This multi-billion dollar industry would never advise that physicians recommend God's natural way of treating illnesses. On the other hand, adequate research, on these natural cures, has not been conducted to apply them to modern day medicine in this country. They should therefore be used as health aids or supplements instead of first line treatments. In time, they may be used as the "drug of choice" for many diseases.

Chapter Twenty Seven

Weight Loss

"When you sit down to eat with a ruler, consider carefully what is before you; and put a knife to your throat if you are a man given to appetite" (Proverbs 23:1-2. Holy Bible, King James Version).

I am often asked what the Bible (or God) has to say about being overweight or obese. Let me assure you that God does not want you to be overweight or obese. Not just so you'll feel better about yourself, but because He loves you, and He doesn't want you to be burdened with the serious health problems that usually accompany these conditions. Our Bibles also teach us that the fruit of the Spirit is love, joy, peace, patience, kindness, goodness, faith, gentleness and self-control. Against such things there is no law (Galatians chapter 5). Christians may fear placing too much emphasis on the physical at the expense of the spiritual, but neglecting your health can be very bad. When we have no control over our eating habits, we lack the self-control that is the fruit of the spirit. We limit our self love, joy, peace, and happiness as well. The key to this situation is a healthy balance. Along with fresh foods, clean waters and air that we cannot see or smell, we also want strong healthy bodies. Without taking care of the physical body, it will be difficult to concern ourselves with the spiritual, yet many of us are either unaware or deny this.

Helping patients lose weight has been one the most enjoyable aspects in my career. That is not to suggest that successfully treating the 45 year old male for his first heart attack or the 80 year old woman for her third stroke doesn't delight me. But, these people already have existing disease. Weight loss treatment can prevent not only strokes or heart attacks, but it also: saves marriages, prevents cancers, unravels metabolic disorders (hypothyroidism, insulin resistance, and diabetes mellitus), prevents blindness, increases job opportunities, saves kidneys, increases one's self-worth and self-esteem, improves fertility, and many other life enhancing states.

On a more personal level, the challenge of successfully fighting obesity brings joy, satisfaction and even hilarity into my life seemingly on a daily basis. Just recently, a 9 year old boy accompanying his mother on her monthly clinic visit displayed concern about his mother's weight loss. After informing her that she has lost a total of fifty pounds, the boy became bewildered. He looked at us as if we were involved in some type of magic trick. He asked: "If my mother lost fifty pounds, what did you do with it? Where did it go? Is it still inside of her? Why can't you find it?"

The American Obesity Association reports the prevalence of obesity to be higher in African-Americans than in Whites and Hispanics. In science, obesity is defined as a body mass index (BMI) greater than 30. A BMI of 25-29.9 indicates that one is overweight. A BMI of 18.5 to 24.9 is normal weight, while less than 18.5 is considered underweight. To determine your BMI, one can use the following formula with your weight in pounds and your height in inches:

$$BMI = \left(\frac{\text{Weight in Pounds}}{(\text{Height in inches})\times(\text{Height in inches})} \right) \times 703$$

BMI	Weight Status
Below 18.5	Underweight
18.5 – 24.9	Normal
25.0 – 29.9	Overweight
30.0 and Above	Obese

For example, a person who weighs 220 pounds and is 6 feet 3 inches (75 inches) tall has a BMI of 27.5.

$$\left(\frac{220 \text{ lbs.}}{(75 \text{ inches}) \times (75 \text{ inches})} \right) \times 703 = 27.5$$

A BMI of 27.5 is indicative of an overweight person (see chart above).

Waist-to-hip ratio

This ratio measures fat distribution and classifies it as gynoid, "hips," or pear obesity. It can also be classified as android, beer belly or apple obesity. Those with such classifications have a higher risk for cardiovascular disease and insulin resistance. A waist circumference of greater than or equal to 40 inches for males and greater than or equal to 35 inches for females also have an increased risk and meets one criteria for the diagnosis of insulin resistance or syndrome X.

Technique for measurements:

Use a non-stretchable measuring tape. Release any twists or kinks in the tape. The tape should touch skin, but never compress the soft tissues. Never take measurements within one hour of a large meal. Measure your waist while in the supine (lying on the back) position as the panniculus (large accumulation of fatty tissue) will shift downward in the standing position. Always began your measurement at the natural waist line. Go midway between the palpated iliac crest (top of the hip bone) and the lowest rib margin. This should fall at the mid-axillary line (just below the center of your under arms). The hip circumference is measured while you are standing erect, arms at the side and feet together. Measure the hips at the maximum circumference over the buttocks. Use the chart below, based on your gender, to determine your health risks.

Eat & Live Longer Waist to Hip Ratio Chart

Male	Female	Health Risk
0.95 or below	0.80 or below	Low Risk
0.96 to 1.0	0.81 to 0.85	Moderate Risk
1.0+	0.85+	High Risk

"The only weight loss plan that is guaranteed to work forever comes from God's dietary laws." R. Eadie, MD.

Chapter Twenty Eight

Exercise

"A man in health, who is both vigorous and his own, should be under no obligatory rules, and have no need, either for a medical attendant, or for a rubber and anointer. His kind of life should afford him variety; he should be now in the country, now in town, and more often about the farm; he should sail, hunt, rest sometimes, but more often take exercise: for whilst inaction weakens the body, work strengthens it; the former brings on premature old age, the latter prolongs youth." A. Cornelius Celsus (ca.10-60)[1]

Exercise, as defined by Hieronymus Mercuralis over 500 years ago, is deliberate and planned movement of the human frame, accompanied by breathlessness and undertaken for the sake of health and fitness. Simply put, exercise means increasing the amount of physical activity more than what our ordinary life demands. Exercise, to our ancestors, was a way of life. As we ran through the tropical forests to capture or avoid animals, demonstrate sportsmanship, climb trees to gather food and swam the tides of deep waters;

we were exercising. The onset of technological advancements created a more sedentary way of life for human beings. Unfortunately, this increase in inactivity also led to an increase in unhealthiness. Fortunately, man has spent the last 50 years developing ways to simulate our daily activity from thousands of years ago. If we knew what exercise did for us, or better yet what the lack of exercise did to us, we might become more active as a people.

Benefits of exercise:

- ✓ Reduces your risk of heart disease, high blood pressure, diabetes, overweight and obesity.
- ✓ Helps you maintain a normal and healthy weight by increasing your metabolism (the rate you burn calories).
- ✓ Keeps joints, tendons and ligaments healthy which improves mobility.
- ✓ Improves sleep.
- ✓ Lowers stress and anxiety.
- ✓ Decreases depression.
- ✓ Increases energy and endurance.
- ✓ Curves appetites and burns calories.

✓ Studies have shown that active women have an approximate 30% reduction in breast cancer risk compared with women who are inactive. Following a breast cancer diagnosis, active breast cancer survivors have reduced risk of breast cancer recurrence and prolonged survival.

✓ Strengthens your heart muscle. A stronger heart can pump more blood with every heartbeat. This means your heart doesn't need to beat as fast during rest or exercise.

✓ Improve blood flow to all parts of your body. A stronger heart muscle pumps blood more efficiently.

✓ Relieves chronic muscle pain and fibromyalgia (chronic and often unexplainable diffuse pain).

✓ Aerobic exercise stimulates the growth of tiny blood vessels (capillaries) in your muscles. This helps your body deliver oxygen to your muscles more efficiently and remove irritating metabolic waste products, such as lactic acid.

✓ Builds strong bones. Weight-bearing aerobic exercise, such as walking, can reduce your risk of osteoporosis and its complications. Low-impact aerobic exercises — such as swimming, cycling and pool exercises — can help keep you fit without putting excessive stress on your joints, making these exercises good choices if you have arthritis.

All forms of increased physical activity will benefit everyone, regardless of your age, gender and past medical history. All exercise programs should begin only after receiving clearance and recommendations from your physician. In particular, you should consult your doctor prior to starting an exercise regimen if you have heart disease, high blood pressure or arthritis and if you ever experienced chest pains or dizziness. Exercise programs should always begin slowly with a gradual increase in intensity and duration.

When developing your exercise regimen, a few things should be considered:

- **Choose an exercise that you will enjoy and that suits you physically**. For example, one with arthritis may choose swimming.
- **Find a partner or a group of people**. Exercising with someone else can make it more enjoyable.
- **Choose a safe and comfortable environment**. When walking, jogging or running, watch out for stray animals and avoid high crime areas. Don't work out too soon after eating or in very hot or cold climates.
- **Don't have the "no pain-no gain" mentally**. While a small amount of soreness is normal after you first start exercising, pain isn't. Stop the exercise if it hurts.
- **Make your workout as fun as possible**. Read, listen to music, talk or watch television while exercising as long as it doesn't interfere with your safety. Find fun things to do like walking

through a zoo, dancing, playing tennis, etc.

- **Be patient**. It can take weeks to months before you notice significant benefits from exercising.
- **Consider keeping an activity log**. Recording your activities allows you to appreciate your progress and vary your exercises.

Where do I begin?

Deciding what exercise to start with is always a challenge. The best answer to the question is: start with exercises that you are sure to do regularly. Spreading out your exercises (throughout the week) yields far greater benefits than doing them in one setting. Also, exercises that increase your heart rate and move large muscles (e.g. arm and leg muscles) are more beneficial.

You should engage in moderate-intensity (e.g. brisk walking, mowing the lawn, dancing, swimming, bicycling) for at least 30 minutes for 5 or more days per week. Eventually, you may want to engage in vigorous-intensity (e.g. heavy yard work, high-impact aerobic dancing, swimming continuous laps, uphill bicycling) physical activity 3 or more days per week for 20 or more minutes per session. Remember, it's never too late to start an active lifestyle. No matter how unfit you look or feel, or how long you have been inactive, research proves that starting a more active lifestyle now will improve your quality of life.

How can I prevent an injury?

You should always start an exercise session with a gradual warm-up period. Take 5-10 minutes to first slowly stretch the muscles you plan to exercise. Then gradually increase the activity of each muscle group. For example, running should always be preceded by brisk walking and then jogging.

After your exercise is complete, allow your muscles to cool down by stretching them again. Always re-stretch the same muscles used in the warm-up. The cool down period should be at least 10-15 minutes long.

The safest way to prevent an injury is to make sure you don't do too much too soon. Always start with an exercise/weight that is fairly easy to you. After your muscles become more familiar with exercise, then gradually increase the intensity. As you increase your activity, start to measure your heart rate (number of heart beats) per minute. Try to keep your heart rate at about 60-85% of your maximum heart rate. This is called your target heart rates.

<u>Maximum heart rate</u> = 220 – your age.

Multiply your maximum heart rate by 0.60 to get the 60% value.

Multiply you maximum heart rate by 0.85 to get the 85% value.

For example, if you are 40 years old, then:

Maximum heart rate = 220 - 40= 180 beats per minute.

60% Target heart rate = 0.60 x 180 = 108 beats per minute.

85% Target heart rate =0.85 x 180 = 153 beats per minute.

When you first start your exercise program, you may want to use the lower number (60%) to calculate your target heart rate. Then, as you're conditioning gradually increases, you may want to use the higher number (85%) to calculate your target heart rate. The range (108-153) is also a good goal for your heart rate. Check your pulse by gently resting your index and middle fingers on the side of your neck (adjacent to your Adam's apple) and counting the beats for 60 seconds. Use a watch with a second hand to time the minute.

What are the best type of exercises to do?

Exercises are essentially broken up into two categories: aerobic (or cardiovascular) and strength training. Aerobic exercise is the type that moves large muscle groups and causes your heart to work harder and pump blood faster while taking deeper breaths. The word *aerobic* refers to improving oxygen consumption within your body. Aerobic exercise helps you live a healthier and longer life. Your body is a complex machine that will get stronger and work more efficiently as it adapts to a regular program of aerobic exercise.

When you're aerobically fit, your body takes in and uses oxygen to sustain movement more efficiently. To do this, your body:

- ❖ **Takes in more oxygen.** You breathe faster and more deeply to maximize the amount of oxygen in your blood stream.
- ❖ **Pumps blood faster and more forcefully.** To produce energy and deliver oxygen more effectively to the rest of your body, your heart beats faster. The force of each beat of your heart increases to maximize blood flow to your muscles and back to your lungs.
- ❖ **Increases the diameter and number of small blood vessels**. To get more oxygen to your muscles, small blood vessels (capillaries) dilate and carry away waste products (e.g. carbon dioxide and lactic acid).

Over time, more capillaries will actually develop in the muscle to provide for more efficient oxygen delivery and waste removal.

* **Avoids overheating.** Your body warms up when you repeatedly move your muscles. To compensate for the rise in temperature, your body releases heat into the air as you breathe out. You also lose heat, water and minerals as you sweat.
* **Releases endorphins.** Regular aerobic exercise releases endorphins which are your body's natural painkillers.

Recommended aerobic exercises:

o **Walking--**This is the most popular form of aerobic exercise. It is simple to do and costs you nothing. Just find yourself a pair of comfortable shoes and walk yourself into a life of health and happiness.
o **Aerobic dancing**
o **Swimming**
o **Bicycling**
o **Cross-country skiing**

- o Running
- o Jogging
- o Aquatic exercise
- o Dancing
- o Stair climbing
- o Elliptical training
- o Rowing

What is strength training exercise?

This type of exercise is important for building strong bones and muscles. It should occupy only about 15-20% of your exercise program. Exercises, like push-ups and lifting weights, are popular strength-training exercises. Make sure to talk to your doctor before beginning them.

For those that find it impossible to start an exercise program or want to simply increase their level of activity, consider the following activities:

- ➢ Walk your (or a neighbor's) dog as often as possible.
- ➢ Walk or bike to nearby stores instead of driving.
- ➢ Do household chores yourself instead of hiring someone or

delegating the duty to other family members.

- ➤ Park farther away at the shopping mall and grocery store and walk the extra distance. Also, never park near the store you plan to visit.
- ➤ Always stand or walk while talking on the phone.
- ➤ Always take a short walk after each meal when possible.
- ➤ Don't use your remote controls on odd numbered months.
- ➤ Always take the stairs instead of the elevator. Or, get off of the elevator a floor early and walk the remainder of the way up.
- ➤ Always pack a jump rope when traveling and do 100 jumps day. Otherwise 100 jumping-jacks will suffice.
- ➤ At work, walk the hallways while conducting small meetings.
- ➤ Schedule exercise time on your calendar and treat it as any other important appointment.
- ➤ Get off of the bus/train a few blocks early and enjoy the extra distance.

Chapter Twenty Nine

Fasting

"But even now," says the Lord, "repent sincerely and return to me with fasting..." (Joel 2:12. Good News Bible, Good News Translation).

The English word "fasting" is derived from the Greek word *nesteia*. Nesteia is a compound of *ne* (a negative prefix) and *esthio* which means "to eat." Hence, the basic root of the word simply means "not to eat." Historically, the first person my research found that participated in abstinence from food for a specific purpose was the biblical prophet named Moses. The ninth chapter of the book of Deuteronomy reminds us that when Moses climbed up the mountain to receive the commandments, he stayed there for forty days and for forty nights without eating or drinking anything.

Fasting is often combined with prayer and represents a spiritual sacrifice while focusing on God and improving your relation with Him. The Old Testament describes a day where God commanded the Israelites to fast. This day was called The Day of Atonement and was the day of confession for previous sins committed. Many people continue to do spiritual fasting while: mourning someone's death, repenting and confessing, in a situation of impending danger, in need of Godly direction and under the instructions of church leaders. Fasting is often done in secret as recommended in Mathew 6:18; *"So that others cannot know that you are fasting-only your Father, who is unseen, will know. And your Father, who sees what you do in private, will reward you"* (Good News Bible, Good News translation).

Fasting has also been incorporated in the lives of many for other reasons. From a nutrition standpoint, fasting is used as a form of cleansing and detoxification. In *Spiritual Nutrition and the Rainbow Diet*, Gabriel Cousens, MD., a California physician and spiritual teacher describes the fasting experience:

> "...fasting in a large context means to abstain from that which is toxic to mind, body, and soul. A way to understand this is that fasting is the elimination of

physical, emotional, and mental toxins from our organism, rather than simply cutting down on or stopping food intake."[1]

From a medical standpoint, fasting is thought to be a method of natural healing. We can appreciate this by observing animals and how they do not eat when they are sick. Conditions for which fasting may be beneficial to man include: colds, flu, environmental allergies, asthma, insomnia, skin diseases, coronary artery disease, angina, bronchitis, headache, constipation, hypertension, diabetes, fatigue, back pain, epilepsy, diarrhea, food allergies, mental illness and obesity.

Every February, since 1999, I have avoided eating chicken, turkey and fish. Incidentally, I have been on a *permanent* beef and pork fast for almost 20 years. My personal experience with fasting has been enlightening. First of all, it allows me to exercise mental strength and discipline. It reminds me of how emotions (e.g. stress) can be misinterpreted as hunger. Differentiating between true hunger and false hunger suddenly becomes obvious. Also, fasting serves as a means of focusing on life challenges that I am faced with. Next, while fasting I feel a sense of rejuvenation. My body feels lighter, well rested and more wholesome. Finally and most importantly, it is act of sacrifice that allows me to commune with God.

To suggest that fasting is perfectly safe would be untrue. The following are some reasons for one to refrain from any fasting activities without a physician's directions:

Diabetes

Underweight
(BMI < 18.5)

Fatigue

Decreased
immune system

Cardiac
Arrhythmias

Cold weather

Pregnancy

Nursing
mothers

Pre & Post-
surgery

Mental illness

Cancers

Peptic Ulcer
Disease

Nutritional
deficiencies

Some enjoy fasting so much that they may overindulge and go beyond the limits. Just like those in the world that are involuntary fasters, depriving yourself of nutrients can lead to disease.

Chapter Thirty

Fruit and Vegetables

"... I am putting you in charge of the fish, the birds, and all the wild animals. I have provided all kinds of grain and all kinds of fruit for you to eat; but for all the wild animals and for all the birds I have provided grass and leafy plants for food ..." (Genesis 1:28-30. Good News Bible. Good News Translation).

I am not sure how you would interpret this scripture, but to me God instructed Adam and Eve to use only grains and fruit as food and nutrition. It was the wild animals and birds that were allowed to eat grass and vegetables. In fact, it wasn't until after Noah and the great flood that He allowed us to extend our diets beyond grains and fruit. This is evident in the ninth chapter of Genesis the second and third verses when God told Noah and his family:

"All the animals, birds, and fish will live in fear of you. They are all placed under your power. Now you can eat them, as well as green plants; I give them all to you for food." (Good News Bible. Good News Translation).

God gave us fruit and vegetables so that we can have fun, tasty and enjoyable foods that prevent and cure diseases. It was His original fast food. The National Institute of Health (NIH) has suggested that we should have at least 5 servings of fruits and vegetables daily. As a people, why are we disobedient to both God and the NIH when it comes to eating our daily intake?

I recommend that all African-American adults consume at least 9 daily servings of fruit and vegetables as our genes have adequately responded to a high amount of fruits and vegetables for thousands of years. We should eat at least 4 servings of fruit and 5 servings of vegetables per day. This way we can reduce or get rid of the diseases that result from not eating enough fruits and vegetables.

Benefits of fruit and vegetables:

- Protect you from diseases (premature aging, cataracts, heart attacks, strokes, kidney disease, cancers, birth defects, high blood pressure and obesity)
- Low in calories
- High in fiber
- Full of vitamins (A&C), minerals, and water
- Contains antioxidants
- Nature's toothbrush

To ensure that you consume 9 servings per day, try:

- Snacking on raw veggies instead of potato chips
- Adding fruit to your (dry) cereal in the morning
- Using the salad bar 100% of the time when dining out
- Drinking pure (unprocessed) juice
- Ordering a veggie pizza and add the meat as an additional topping

Don't forget what constitutes a serving:

- ½ cup of fresh, frozen or canned fruits or vegetables
- 1 cup of raw leafy greens
- ¾ cup (6 oz) of fruit or vegetable juice
- 1 medium-size piece of fruit
- ½ cup of peas or cooked dry beans
- ¼ cup of dried fruit

Fruit and vegetables that are high in Vitamin A include:

Apricots, cantaloupe, carrots, kale, collards, leaf lettuce, mango, romaine lettuce, spinach, sweet potato, winter squash (acorn, hubbard)

Fruits and vegetables that are high in vitamin C include:

apricots, broccoli, brussels sprouts, cabbage, cantaloupe, cauliflower, chili peppers, collards, grapefruit, honeydew melon, kiwi fruit, mango, mustard greens, orange, orange juice, pineapple, plum, potato with skin, spinach, strawberries, bell peppers, tangerine, tomatoes, watermelon

Fruits and vegetables that are good sources of fiber include:

apples, bananas, blackberries, blueberries, brussels sprouts, carrots, cherries, cooked beans and peas (kidney, navy, lima, and pinto beans, lentils, black-eyed peas), dates, figs, grapefruit, kiwi fruit, orange, pear, prunes, raspberries, spinach, strawberries, sweet potato

There is a misperception in our community that purchasing fruit and vegetables is not affordable. The truth of the matter is that they are actually good buys. Considering that they are vitamin and nutrient dense and promote healthy and longer lives should spark your interest in comparing prices. What should they be compared to? They should be compared to the foods we often eat in place of them. This includes your cookies, chips, candy and other junk foods. If potato chips usually cost you about 50 cents for a small (single serving) bag, compare that to a 20 cent banana. Or compare a 65 cent pack of cookies to a 15 cent apple.

Chapter Thirty One

Understanding Nutritional Facts Labels

"Study to show thyself approved unto God, a workman that needeth not to be ashamed, rightly dividing the word of truth." (II Timothy 2:15. Holy Bible, King James Version).

Before you begin reading this chapter, I suggest that you grab a couple of your favorite packaged or canned food items as a reference.

For many of us, understanding how to interpret Nutrition Facts labels is a task. Not knowing the "facts" about the foods you put into your body is nothing short of foolish. Most of the information you need to know is provided to you, by the Federal Government, on the back of each food item. Since the Government has done their job, being able to understand what is listed is your job. In the 1970's, food manufacturers were using arbitrary labels on their foods items. In the early 1990's, the Nutrition Labeling and Education Act (NLEA) was initiated and the FDA mandated labeling on all foods with the exception of meat and poultry which was being regulated by the USDA (you should ask yourself why there is no labeling for meat).

In 1994, Nutrition Facts labels became mandatory and standardized. The labels were based on a 2,000 calorie diet directed to those over 4 years of age. This large caloric amount was thought to be the average American daily caloric intake. Its purpose was to list major components of each food item, bad or good, so that the consumer had a better idea of what he or she was eating and could better choose which foods they should eat.

The U.S. government now requires that all packaged food products contain the following information:

- Nutrition Facts and ingredient list
- The common name of the product
- Weight, measure or count of net contents
- Name, address and (optional) e-mail address of the manufacturer

Before we go any further, it is important to note the following caloric equivalents:

- 1 gram of fat = 9 calories
- 1 gram of protein = 4 calories
- 1 gram of carbohydrates = 4 calories
- 1 gram of alcohol = 7 calories

Follow these steps when reading the nutrition Facts labels:

1. **Serving Size**: The first place you should look is at the serving size and the number of servings in the package. These are standardized into familiar units (i.e. cups and pieces) and the metric amount (i.e. grams).
2. **Servings Per Container**: Below the serving size are the servings per container. Always look at the serving size as **the number of people that should be eating this entire item**. This value is very important because if you eat the whole item by yourself, you may need to make adjustments to all of the numbers indicated below. For example, if the total number of calories per serving is 200 and

the serving size is 2, then eating the whole package by yourself means that you will be consuming a total of 400 calories (200 calories x 2 servings). You must also multiply all of the other numerical values (total fat, cholesterol, sodium, carbohydrates, protein, etc.) x 2 (for a 2 serving package) if you eat the entire package.

3. **Calories**: The calories are listed in two ways on packaged foods. (1) Total calories and (2) calories from fat. The calories provide a measure of how much energy you get from a serving. You must pay great attention to the calorie listing when it comes to managing your weight. Remember these three important points: **3,500 calories = 1 pound, the number of servings you consume determines the number of calories you actually eat (your portion amount) and more than 300 calories (per serving) is too much.** In order to lose 1 pound per week, simply reduce your daily caloric intake by 500. African Americans consume

more calories than needed and often fall short of the nutrients needed.

4. **Nutrients**: The next section describes the nutrients in the packaged food. There are certain nutrients that must always be listed because they negatively affect the health of many Americans (especially African Americans), those nutrients include carbohydrates, sugar and protein. Remember: **these nutrients must be limited.** Other nutrients (fiber, vitamins A and C, calcium and iron) are the nutrients that you want to consume plenty of. A deficiency of any of these leads to disease.

5. The bottom of the label is a footnote that must be used in correlation with the right column of the label under the heading "% Daily Value." (DV) Notice that the percent daily value is based on a 2,000 calorie diet and that your daily value may be higher or lower depending on your caloric needs. You and I both know that your daily caloric intake should be less than 2,000

calories and probably right around 1,000. If this is the case, you should double the % daily value of each nutrient since your daily caloric intake is ½ of the 2,000. As a rule of thumb, a % DV of 5% or less is low and 20% or more is high. Apply these values to the nutrient scores. A good product has a %DV of fiber, vitamin A, vitamin C, calcium, protein and iron that is 20% or greater. A good item also has a % DV of fat (total, Trans and saturated), cholesterol, sodium, sugar and total carbohydrates that is 5% or less.

An uneducated consumer looks at the brand and the price of an item when shopping. A smart consumer looks at the brand, the nutrition facts label, the price of the item and then compares it to other brands before making the healthiest choice. As an educated shopper, master the nutrition facts label and teach it to your children, family, friends and community.

Chapter Thirty Two

The Eat Right - Sunlight Theory

The Introduction

"On the day that the Lord gave the men of Israel victory over the Amorites, Joshua spoke to the Lord. In the presence of the Israelites he said, "Sun, stand still over Gibeon..." (Joshua 10:12. Good News Bible, Good News Translation).

Then God commanded, "Let lights appear in the sky to separate day from night and to show the time when days, years, and religious festivals begin; they will shine in the sky to give light to the earth" – and it was done. So God made the two larger lights, the sun to rule over the day and the moon to rule over the night; he also made the stars. He placed the lights in the sky to shine on the earth, to rule over the day and the night, and to separate light from darkness. And God was pleased with what he saw. Evening passed and morning came – that was the fourth day (Genesis 1:14-19. Good News Bible, Good News Translation).

Africans have appreciated the relationship between man and the sun for thousands of years. The sun is the primary energy source for this energized planet we call the earth. This big bright heavenly body provides a great energy that is indispensable to all nature. This is why the earth moves faster when it is nearest the sun and slower when it is farthest from the sun. Humanity gets a great deal of its vitality, joy, peace and happiness from the sun. Sunlight was used to prevent and treat the diseases of ancient Africans for many years before Egypt's advanced civilization came. It is responsible for blowing winds, ocean currents and water flow, oil, the development of natural gases and maintaining all life forms on earth.

Through nature, God has devised a way to transfer this energy from a star with a diameter of 864,938 miles (109 times the size of the earth) and a location over 91 million miles away to the many microscopic cells found within living matter here on earth. Amazing! Just like planets and animals, the sun is made of a predominant element called hydrogen. The sun's hydrogen atoms fuse together and create helium. This fusion creates the energy that is radiated to us in the form of sunlight. This sunlight is captured here on earth by the plant life. Only plants (and algae) can convert this sunlight energy into food energy. In my mind, this is why God made the sun, the waters and the plants before making animals and man. Man, in turn, gets their share of sunlight energy by eating the energized plants. It is no coincidence that plants and man are in the upright position for the majority of their lifespan. Any non-scientific person could figure out that this is because the sun sits high above them in the sky. We naturally grow upward or vertically (instead of outward or horizontally) towards this great source of power created by our God.

The energy emitted from the sun is transferred to plants by a process called photosynthesis. The prefix *photo* refers to the sunlight energy and *synthesis* means the ability to make food energy. For photosynthesis to occur plants need sunlight energy, water and a gas called carbon dioxide. Nearly everything that we interact with is composed of Hydrogen (H), Carbon (C), and Oxygen

(O) atoms. These atoms can fuse together to form molecules. For example, if two hydrogen atoms plus an oxygen atom fuse, they form water (H+H+O=H2O=Water). Or, if a carbon atom joins water, it makes sugar (C+H2O=CH2O=Sugar). A final example would be how a carbon atom and two oxygen atoms make carbon dioxide (C+O+O=CO2=Carbon dioxide). To fuse these atoms together to make such molecules, energy must be added. This energy comes from the sunlight. Conversely, breaking a molecule (e.g. Sugar/CH2O) down into individual atoms produces energy.

When the leaves of a corn plant interact with carbon dioxide and water in the presence of sunlight energy, it produces sugar (C02+H2O=CH2O/Sugar with two oxygen atoms (02) remaining. These two oxygen atoms are released into the air by the plants for man to breathe. This is how a plant's sugar molecule is stored as sunlight energy. When man eats the ear of the sweet corn, his body breaks those sugar molecules apart to get the energy back out. This is the energy that allows man to walk, talk, run, hunt, gather, think, see and grow.

Because God's perfect system works as a continuous cycle, man must give this energy back to the environment. To get the energy out of the sugar, our bodies must turn it back in to water and carbon dioxide, just as it started. The process begins when man breaths in the oxygen molecules (02) that we got from the plant's photosynthesis. This Oxygen molecule binds to the sugar molecule to produce water and carbon dioxide (02 + CH20 = C02 + H20). The carbon dioxide is the food for the plant.

Man, plants, and animals continuously exchange oxygen, carbon dioxide and water. Through this cycle, all living things on earth are related and working harmoniously as one. Man and animals make carbon dioxide for plants, and plants make oxygen for man and animals. The sun provides the energy to get this process started and continue the cycle.

Another function of the sun is to provide light as well as enlightenment for man. In a nonphysical sense, this light allows us to clearly see (understand) many things, including when to eat. It also energizes our brain, moods and metabolism. How? The sun positively affects the sum of man's physical and chemical processes by which its material substance is produced, maintained, and destroyed, and by which his body's energy is made available (i.e. man's metabolism). First of all, man should eat when the sun is visible or provides light for the outdoors. On the other hand, man should not eat when the sun is not visible or when the earth is void of sunlight. During daylight and sun exposure, man is most active and the metabolism of man is operating at its maximum point...Eat right, sunlight! During sunlight exposure, you have an increase in your:

1. **Metabolism,** so you are more likely to burn the food you ate and less likely to store the food you ate (as fat). The energy in is more likely to be equal to the energy out yielding no net gain of calories.

2. **Digestion,** so you have optimal function of your chew-digest-absorb-utilize-excrete cycle. Your heart rate increases, which burns

calories and sends adequate blood to your brain and muscles.

3. **Respirations**, allows improvement of the oxygen-carbon dioxide exchange system. Your body tissues receive more oxygen and get rid of the carbon dioxide.

4. **Serotonin**, (a chemical made in the central nervous system and gastrointestinal tract) which decreases hunger and makes it less likely for one to overeat.

5. **Energy level**, because of a decrease in melatonin (a hormone produced in the brain from the amino acid tryptophan).

As the sun's radiant energy level decreases with sunset, the rate of the metabolic processes within man decreases as well. This includes your ability to digest your food properly and burn any of the consumed calories. If man consumes an excess of calories during this period of absent sunlight, he is most likely to store the food energy as fat. Therefore, no or a very small amount of healthy, and very low calorie foods must be eaten after the sun has set. This should preferably include herbal drinks such as green, black or white tea, a small amount of protein and no sugar. Without sunlight, your body goes into the "save energy" mode. All of your bodily functions slow down so you don't need the "day-light" amount of energy.

During the lack of sunlight exposure, you will have a significant <u>decrease</u> in your:

1. **Metabolism,** so you are more likely to store the calories (as fat) you eat instead of burn them. This will always lead to weight gain.

2. **Digestion,** so your food is less likely to be adequately utilized. It will have a longer passage time inside of your intestines. This would lead to constipation, toxin build-up, and weight gain.

4. **Heart rate,** so blood flow to major organs decreases.

5. **Respirations,** since your body needs less oxygen in this sun-free mode.

6. **Activity**, as sluggishness is a result of the type of foods eaten and the increase in melatonin. Sunset is time for rest and rejuvenation.

I was fortunate to visit Torino Italy in February 2006 for the Winter Olympics. The Italians, I noticed, were rather lean or certainly not suffering from obesity the way Americans do. I also recognized that their largest consumption of food (calories) took place when the sun was at its highest peak. That is, at noon day. Dinner, to them, was a small healthy meal coinciding with the setting of the sun. They follow God's nature and it shows as they have healthier hearts than most Americans.

During colder seasons, man should eat even less when it is day light. In the northern hemisphere, the winter solstice is the day of the year (near December 22) when the sun is farthest south. The winter solstice is the shortest day of the year, in the sense that the length of time elapsed between sunrise and sunset on this day is a minimum for the year, hence so should your caloric intake. Also, the sun warms the body as it transfers its energy to man. Our bodies must maintain a certain body temperature for our cells to work properly, so in turn we must release any extra energy back into our environment. To do so, our heart rate and other bodily functions increase. This burns calories, rids fat and produces a healthier and leaner body.

We can look at another aspect of the relationship between the sun and plants as a confirmation of my "eat right-sunlight" theory. Plants produce energies during the day light as it networks with the sun. Once the sunlight is no longer available to the plants, they use the energy to grow and prepare for the next day's exposure. We must do the same by eating when we can maximize our energy expenditure. Increase your caloric intake as the sun rises above us in the sky, and decrease your caloric intake as the sun lowers itself before vanishing. Once the sun is gone from the sky for the day, all living things should stop eating. Just as nature would have it, thousands of years ago, man experienced winters with long nights and little food, and summers with short nights and an abundance of food.

Animals are very aware of the cycles of God and the importance of the sun. Although roosters may crow throughout the entire cycle of the day, they make it a point to crow loudly at the time when half of the sun has risen above the horizon. This thunderous sound of rejoicing and rejuvenation symbolizes the restart of the cycle of the day and the Eat Right-Sunlight process.

A 24-hour biological clock is found in all plants and animals. It is known as the circadian rhythm (or circadian cycle). It was believed, by primitive man, that the sun told them when they were to eat and when they were to sleep. Today, the circadian cycle is also known to influence the sleeping and feeding patterns of all animals, especially human beings. What is the link?

The circadian rhythm is a 24-hour cycle of the functions found in all living beings. In fact, the term "circadian," so named by Franz Halberg, is Latin translation for "circa" and "dies" which literally means "about a day." This cycle is controlled by the presence or absence of the sun. Solar energy is transferred to brain energy which influences sleep, hunger, metabolism and other bodily functions. As soon as man exposes himself to sunlight, the transformation begins:

1. Sun energy interacts with the light receptors in the retina (the innermost coat of the posterior part of the eyeball).
2. This energy is then transferred to the hypothalamus via the retinohypothalamic tract.
3. The light information is then given to the suprachiasmatic nucleus (SCN) of the hypothalamus.
4. From the SCN, the impulses are spread along the pineal nerve to the pineal gland.

The pineal gland, like the retina, has light receptors. It was called "the third eye" by ancient Africans. It is represented on the back of the U.S. dollar bill as the eye atop the pyramid of the great seal. The pineal gland works in harmony with the hypothalamus gland, directing the body's hunger, thirst, sleep-wake cycle, sexual desire and the biological clock that determines our aging process. It is in essence of the body's internal clock and the force behind the circadian cycle. Sun exposure (or stimulation of the pineal gland) results in the decrease in melatonin production and an increase in serotonin production. This low level of melatonin increases metabolism, decreases sleepiness, provides alertness, energizes, stimulates the brain, and stimulates the appetite as needed. In the absence of sunlight, melatonin production is increased. High melatonin levels make man feel tranquil, relaxed, calm, sedate and sleepy.

Serotonin is another very important and mystifying chemical that is also produced by the pineal gland. Most of our serotonin is produced in the early morning, when God's first rays of sunshine stimulate the pineal gland and it converts the amino acid tryptophan (found heavily in turkey meat) into serotonin. High blood levels of serotonin suppress hunger, reverse depression (mode of action for antidepressant drugs), provides satiety (fullness sensation) and relieves certain pains such as migraine and tension headaches. Again, during the hours of darkness, the pineal gland is stimulated to produce melatonin (the sleep hormone) from a hopefully adequate supply of this serotonin.

The fact that serotonin improves one's mood offers explanation as to why we crave certain "comfort" foods when we feel stressed, lonely, sad and depressed. We distinctively desire foods high in tryptophan hoping to elevate our serotonin levels. In states where sunlight exposure is limited throughout several months of the year (i.e. Michigan, Illinois, New York), you will notice a high rate of obesity as a result of over indulgence in such foods. A substantial amount of these foods is needed to produce a significant amount of serotonin. These foods are often high in sugar, fat and unnecessary calories. Comfort foods that are often abused and that are high in tryptophan include:

- Ice cream
- Fruit Pies
- Cake
- Cookies
- Dairy products: cheese, milk, etc.
- Rice
- Pasta
- Pastries

- Soy products (milk, tofu and nuts)
- Probably your favorite junk food when you feel down

Eating, as you now understand, should be done during hours of sun exposure. Research has shown that people can suffer from a disorder called night eating syndrome. This disease can lead to being overweight, obese and/or depressed. Night eating syndrome is present when a person eats after the sun sets. Night eaters have the following characteristics:

- Eat little or have no appetite before sun set.

- Eating more food after sunset than before sun set.

- Eating more than half of daily food intake after sunset.

- Awaken throughout the night from sleep and must eat in order to fall back asleep.

The next time you consider a vacation, ask yourself why you want to spend it in an environment with an excessive amount of sunlight. Not only does it give you an inexplicable degree of energy, it enlightens you. We have gotten away from utilizing the many benefits of the sun.

Man's earliest means of tracking the movement of the sun, as it relates to time, was with the creation of the sundial. The Egyptians and subsequently the ancient Chaldeans mastered the sundial. Biblically speaking (2 Kings, 20:1-11), when King Hezekiah had fallen sick and was told by the prophet that he was to prepare for his death. He prayed to God for a longer life. God heard his prayer and sent Isaiah to explain to him how to heal himself of his illness. King Hezekiah wanted a sign from God to assure him of his full recovery and his ability to return to the temple in a 3 day period. God told him that he would move King Ahaz's sundial back ten degrees as a sign of his promise to allow him to live fifteen years longer and return to the temple.

The process of tracking time with sundials to determine when one should eat, instead of using the circadian cycles, was not accepted by many during those days. For centuries this was debated by many philosophers and healers as new sickness began to appear among the people. Plautus expressed his concerns in 200 BCE when he said:

"The gods confound the man who first found out how to distinguish hours. Confound him, too! Who in this place set up a sundial to cut and hack my days so wretchedly into small pieces! When I was a boy, my belly was my sundial - one more sure, truer, and more exact than any of them. This dial told me when 'twas proper time to go to dinner, when I had ought to eat. But nowadays, why even when I have, I can't fall to unless the inhabitants, shrunk up with hunger, creep along the streets."[1]

Sunlight provides nourishment and energy for all living things. It regulates the temperature and humidity of the earth's atmosphere, keeping it at life-supporting levels. It initiates rain and snow and replenishes our rivers and lakes. All food we eat has a relationship to sunlight. These are some other benefits of sunlight:

- Produces vitamin D
- Decreases blood cholesterol
- Decreases blood sugar
- Kills germs, disinfects
- Increases aerobic fitness
- Increases alertness, energy, and enthusiasm
- Promotes a feeling of well being

"Truly the light is sweet, and a pleasant thing it is for the eyes to behold the sun." (Ecclesiastes 11:7. Holy Bible, King James Version). Could this scripture have the benefits of the SCN of the hypothalamus in mind?

Chapter Thirty Three

Substitutions to Live Longer

"None of us hate our bodies. Instead, we feed them, and take care of them...," (Ephesians 5:29. Good News Bible, Good News Translation).

Choosing a new way of eating is like choosing a new of life. My recommendations of what to eat are based on scientific evidence, medical research, personal experience and common sense. The most challenging aspect of dietary modifications is how to substitute your present "bad choices" with your future "good choices."

Salt

Salt! Salt! Salt! The flavorsome enemy of the African-American! We have been conditioned to accept salt as a taste enhancer ideal for the improvement of our already greasy, fat ridden and low-in-nutrient foods. Salt single handedly has caused more disease than any other combination of minerals know to man. Because of its "salty" taste, it has now become a part of the Africa-American culture. Today's soul food restaurants would not dare have it absent from one of its dining tables.

Some of us are unaware of the variety salts and how they can produce at least five) different taste sensations: salty (sodium chloride); sweet (lead diacetate); sour (potassium bitartrate); bitter (magnesium sulfate); and umami or savory (monosodium glutamate). We simply enjoy the sensation we experience when we shower our chow with these small white crystals that lead to our high blood pressure, swelling, heart attacks, strokes and kidney failure.

The first documentation of salt production was (you guessed it) in Africa. Salt had its beginning around 4000 B.C., in Egypt, and later in Greece and Rome. Salt was very valuable and used to preserve and eventually to flavor foods. In Ancient Rome, salt started to be used as money, originating the current Latin-derivative word we commonly use; *salary*. Generally, payments to Roman workers were made in the form of salt. Until about the 18th century, salt was also given to the parents of the groom in marriage.

Unfortunately for those paid with salt, it was easily ruined by rain and other factors.

But salt is not the 'be all to end all' additive for food. Salt can be substituted with fresh garlic powder, nutmeg, lemon juice, cinnamon, flavored vinegar, cumin, fresh ground pepper, tarragon, oregano, lime juice, powdered onion, cayenne pepper, chili powder, black pepper, ground cloves, ground allspice, celery seeds, coriander seeds and ground cardamom seeds.

Getting patients to accept the reality that adding salt to your food is both unhealthy and unnecessary is always a difficult task for health care providers within the Africa-American community. For me, convincing health care providers that salt substitutes (e.g. potassium chloride salts) can also be detrimental to their patients is an even greater challenge. For example, people with kidney disease, pregnancy, stomach ulcers, diarrhea and Addison's disease should use potassium chloride and other salt substitutes with caution. They can also cause the following side effects: chest pains, irregular heartbeats, confusion, weakness or paralysis, stomach pains or cramping, rash, anxiety, numbness and tingling. Finally, certain medications cannot be used with potassium chloride (e.g. certain non-steroidal anti-inflammatory drugs such as Motrin, prednisone, diuretics, beta blockers, as well as, prednisone, diuretics, beta blockers and ace-inhibitors).

Soft Drinks (a.k.a. Soda, Soda, Pop)

Regardless of how you refer to this drink containing carbonated water and artificial flavorings, you have got to stop drinking it. If you are in need of weight loss and find it very difficult to stop consuming caffeine, you may want to consider temporarily switching to diet soda. Otherwise, stick to drinks that have some nutritious value. A good habit to develop is preparing your daily drinks from whole fruits and vegetables. Using a household blender or juicer is a quick and simple way to prepare natural fluids for your consumption.

The ideal substitution for all drinks would be water. This natural hydrator should be consumed first and foremost; at least 64 ounces per day. Fruits and vegetables can be added to water in order to provide flavor and sweetness the natural way. Fruit juices that are unsweetened and with no added preservatives (100%) can be used but should be used with caution especially if you are attempting to lose weight. They should be limited to 16 ounces daily. To prevent rapid blood sugar elevations and provide more natural fruit flavored drinks, dilute your 16 ounces of juice with water to help increase your daily consumption. In most cases, you won't notice a significant difference in taste.

Sugar

First of all, many physicians and medical publications deny that sugar causes diabetes and simply consider this a myth. I beg to differ. If you research causes of insulin resistance, a precursor to diabetes, you will find the following:

- Abdominal obesity: a waist circumference over 102 cm (40 in) in men and over 88 cm (35 inches) in women.
- Elevated serum triglycerides (150 mg/dl or above).
- Elevated HDL cholesterol (40mg/dl or lower in men and 50mg/dl or lower in women).
- Blood pressure of 130/85 or more.
- Fasting blood glucose of 110 mg/dl or above (some groups say 100mg/dl).

Please believe, if you consume too much sugar, you will at least develop abdominal obesity, insulin resistance and finally diabetes. Not only diabetes, but sugar consumption can lead to many other diseases. The consumption of even naturally concentrated sugars of any nature (honey, maple sugar, date sugar, etc.) must be limited.

God also gave us access to sugars in the fruit and vegetables he surrounded us with. Your sugar substitutions should begin here. In addition to fruits, consider the following: stevia powder, mashed bananas, apple butter, apple sauce, plum butter, orange squash, ginger spice, nutmeg, cloves, vanilla spice or cinnamon spice. You may want to consider heating of cooking with fruit as it makes the fruit taste much sweeter.

Butter, Margarine and other Fats

I know cooking without some type of fat seems virtually impossible. Try using flaxseed oil, canola oil, olive oil, avocado oil, walnut oil or even mustard oil. Challenge yourself by eliminating the butter, lard, margarine and shortening for 30 days. This will show you that you really can live without them.

To improve the Omega-6 to Omega-3 fat ratio, consider combining some of these alternative oils. For example, consider mixing those with good Omega-6 to Omega-3 fat ratios (flaxseed, canola or mustard) with those of not as good ratios (olive and avocado). Your other option would be to use olive oil with cooking and simply take your daily omega-3 oil supplements. Remember to stay away from the oils with poor

Omega-6 to Omega-3 fat ratios such as: coconut, corn, peanut, sunflower, etc.

Regardless of what you choose, you should avoid butter as much as possible. The new margarines now with trans-fats may be a healthier way to go but must be limited as well. Once again, fruit substitutes are always an option. Check out the fruit spreads or preserves with extra fruit and no added sugars.

Alcohol

"And the Lord spoke to Moses, saying, Speak to the children of Israel, and say to them: 'When either a man or a woman consecrates an offering to take the vow of a Nazirite, to separate himself to the Lord, he shall separate himself from wine and strong drink..." (Numbers 6:1-4. Holy Bible, King James Version).

Past day Africans used wine for medicinal purposes such as for the treatment of headaches, anxiety, insomnia, digestive problems and some cardiac abnormalities. When used only occasionally and responsibly, alcohol can provide many health benefits. Enjoying an alcoholic beverage along with dinner dates back many years before Jesus did so during the last supper. Wine contains both phytochemicals and antioxidants, both of which are life promoting substances. When used as a marinate and meat tenderizer, wine can add life to the flavor of your meats. Just make sure you choose a wine with no added salt. Wine can also be added to cooked dishes to exacerbate or deepen tastes already present.

Any male that consumes more than two (females more than one) alcoholic beverages daily should seek immediate attention for over consumption. This amount of alcohol can lead to alcoholism and other serious health problems. No substitute for over consumption of alcohol is recommended until a trained clinician evaluates and treats you. Even with the use of non-alcoholic beers, a professional should be involved as this practice has proven to not cure alcoholism exclusively. This is true in part because non-alcoholic beers are very low alcoholic beverages. They have an alcohol content of less than 1/2 of 1%

by volume but none of the beers are completely alcohol free.

Juice/Fruit

Fruit juice for you or children is by no means the healthiest drink to consume. In comparison to eating whole fruit, juice is not a good choice. Why? Because juice is a processed product and it is more rapidly digested than the whole fruit. This means that the glycemic index of the fruit juice will be higher than the parent fruit. Also a glass of juice has almost three times as many calories than does the whole fruit. Finally, the whole fruit contains fiber and minerals that aren't found in the juice. One solution to this problem is to use a juicer so that you and your family can enjoy "God's fruit juice" full of his sugar, vitamins, minerals and fiber.

Bread

White bread is a "no-no" because it is made from bleached flour. Also because this flour is void of the nutrients and because your body quickly converts it to sugar. If you find it a must to eat bread, then you should only eat whole wheat or whole-grain high-fiber breads. In fact, you should choose 100% stone-ground whole wheat or whole-grain high-fiber bread. Make sure than each slice has between 2 and three grams of fiber and try eat only one slice per day.

Vinegar

For those that do not appreciate the unique taste of vinegars, it can be replaced with lime or lemon juice. Usually, recipes that are tomato based with vinegar (e.g. salsa) use lime juice. Fruit recipes that require the addition of vinegar will taste just fine if lemon juice is used instead.

Dairy

I have made it clear that I greatly oppose milk consumption and believe that other dairy products should be used only sparingly. Most cheeses should be avoided since, as you now know, they are high in saturated fat. If cheese is a must for you, focus on the nonfat options (e.g. nonfat cream cheese), feta or stilton. Even with these, you should try your best to use them as little as possible.

Tea and Coffee

Tea is the caffeinated drink of choice and should replace coffee. Try black tea instead of coffee. If coffee is your thing, drink decaffeinated. Like your strong black skin, coffee should be left that way. Adding sugar and dairy creams to your coffee only adds calories.

Burgers

Beef burgers are a taboo item. Your burgers from this point on should be made from ground chicken or turkey meat. You should get rid of the bun, forget about the bacon and use low calorie toping only. Make sure to include your raw vegetables (lettuce, tomatoes, onions, pickles).

Rice

White rice is bad rice. Instead, eat long grain, brown, wild or basmati since they have a lower GI thus taking longer to break down then white rice. They should still be limited.

Dessert

You must "desert the dessert." Focus on eating sweet fruit in lieu of the sweets. Treat yourself to an occasional dessert but make sure that it's worth eating it. You must subconsciously place a price tag on these types of foods. Ask yourself: "is it really worth the calories." You can help yourself with an answer to this question by considering how common the dessert is. Your grandmother's homemade cherry pie that you taste only once a year may be worth it. Vanilla ice cream from the local parlor certainly is not and should be passed up every time.

Water

No substitute exists. Remember to drink a glass of water before each meal. In fact, you should probably put this book down and enjoy a tall of water right about now. (I can't believe you even looked to see what I would suggest to take the place of the most abundant matter in your body!)

Cereals

Sugar coated, processed, character related cereals usually do more damage and are nutritionally just as bad as candy. Do you approve of giving your child candy for breakfast? The sugar load within the cereal and milk is horrendous and must be eliminated from our children's diet.

Consider using high fiber, whole-grain, large flake cold cereals instead. The fiber content is most important and should be at least 10 grams per serving. To this, fruit, nuts and yogurt can be added. Adults and children can eat this en route to work or school in the morning to get the day started off right. Many are surprised to discover how much sugar and milk is not needed. Heated oatmeal prepared with water is the ideal warm cereal. Oat bran and oat meal have low Glycemic Indices and therefore will keep your stomach full longer. Other benefits include keeping your blood pressure and cholesterol lower. Again, fruit can be added to satisfy your sugar needs.

Chapter Thirty Four

Six Steps to Successful Eating and Living Longer

1. Learn your ideal weight. Get there and stay there.

And Joab said to Amasa, Art thou in health, my brother? (2 Samuel 20:9. Holy Bible, King James Version).

Ideal body weights have been debated for years. It never really made much of a difference until recently, when America (and now the rest of the world) began to suffer from overweight and obesity. Although less accurate than BMI, the ideal body weight of an individual has also been determined based on the height (in feet inches) and the size of the body frame (small, medium and large) in comparison to the rates of morbidity and mortality.

Your body frame can be determined by referencing your wrist. Use your dominant middle finger and thumb and wrap them around your non-dominant wrist as tightly as tolerable. Be sure to wrap them around the thinnest part of your wrist. You have a small frame if the fingers overlap. If the fingers barely touch, you have a medium sized frame. Those with large frames find that their dominant thumb and index fingers do not touch.

Ideal Body Weight for Women

Height in Feet Inches	Small Frame	Medium Frame	Large Frame
4' 10"	102-111	109-121	118-131
4' 11"	103-113	111-123	120-134
5' 0"	104-115	113-126	122-137
5' 1"	106-118	115-129	125-140
5' 2"	108-121	118-132	128-143
5' 3"	111-124	121-135	131-147
5' 4"	114-127	124-138	134-151
5' 5"	117-130	127-141	137-155
5' 6"	120-133	130-144	140-159
5' 7"	123-136	133-147	143-163
5' 8"	126-139	136-150	146-167
5' 9"	129-142	139-153	149-170
5' 10"	132-145	142-156	152-173
5' 11"	135-148	145-159	155-176
6' 0"	138-151	148-162	158-179

African-American men often find it hard to accept their recommended ideal body weight. For example, explaining to a 6 feet tall 36 year old non-athletic African-American male of large framing that his 210 pound weight is unacceptable could be problematic. These weights at ages 25-59 are based on the lowest level of sickness and death and are according to frame sizes. If not weighed in the nude, 5 pounds should be subtracted for clothing. Shoes should be removed during weigh-ins.

Ideal Body Weight for Men

Height Feet Inches	Small Frame	Medium Frame	Large Frame
5' 2"	128-134	131-141	138-150
5' 3"	130-136	133-143	140-153
5" 4"	132-138	135-145	142-156
5' 5"	134-140	137-148	144-160
5' 6"	136-142	139-151	146-164
5' 7"	138-145	142-154	149-168
5' 8"	140-148	145-157	152-172
5' 9"	142-151	148-160	155-176
5' 10"	144-154	151-163	158-180
5' 11"	146-157	154-166	161-184
6' 0"	149-160	157-170	164-188
6' 1"	152-164	160-174	168-192
6' 2"	155-168	164-178	172-197
6' 3"	158-172	167-182	176-202
6' 4"	162-176	171-187	181-207

Please take these recommendations seriously and reduce your weight as needed. Weighing yourself every Sunday morning can help you better plan your weekly meals. Choosing the proper food groups while maintaining proper caloric intake to stay at your ideal body weight is paramount.

Of course, you have to make your own decisions about your life and your health and refusing to comply is your prerogative. But, for the sake of your health and life longevity, noncompliance is not advised. If you refuse to or are unable to reduce your weight to the recommended level, at least try to get to a level 10-20% above the maximum limit. Remember, the weight you want isn't necessarily the weight you need. It's all about your health and reducing your risk factors of life threatening disease.

2. **Learn your family medical history**.

"Is there no medicine in Gilead? Are there no doctors there? Why, then, have my people not been healed"? (Jeremiah 8:22. Good News Bible, Good News Translation).

My answer to this biblical question is because people refuse to eat the God-given and mandated foods that will prolong their life spans.

Contrary to what you believe, the many health forms you are required to complete and the endless questions you are asked during your medical 'interrogation' help your physician tremendously. Now, it's time for you to begin helping yourself. What I am recommending is that you devise a thorough medical history of your family that extends at least three generations in your past. This should include the health problems of your siblings, aunts, uncles, grandparents, great aunts, great uncles and your great-grandparents. Be sure to indicate the age at which each deceased died, and the respective illnesses they had.

Like your physician, you should pay close attention to the type of diseases, age of onset of diseases, patterns of diseases, and the genders affected. With this valuable information, you can almost predict what illness you will suffer from if you live a similar lifestyle to your older family members. For example, if both of your parents developed hypertension in their forties, there is a strong possibility that you will too, unless you change your lifestyle (eating to live longer, exercise regularly, relieve stresses, etc.). If you make these changes, you would be more likely to become educated on the causes, effects and preventions of hypertension. You would also be more likely to have your blood pressure checked regularly and be compliant if prescribed medications.

Your family medical history should be reviewed and updated at least annually. The beginning of every year is an ideal time to do this. This is a time when many family members get together for the holidays. Or, you can always include it in your New Year's resolution. Another great time to develop or revise your family medical history information is during a family reunion. This point is so extremely important that "family health" should be added to your family reunion agenda of activities. Why not be the one to lead the charge to collect data from interested family members and distributing a summary of results following the reunion? You and your family could live longer by simply being prepared and armed with understanding of which diseases you may be faced with.

3. Change your way of thinking and your choice of foods.

"When I was a child, I spoke like a child; I thought like a child, I reasoned like a child. When I became a man, I gave up childish ways." (1 Corinthians 13:11. The Holy Bible, The New English Standard Version Translation).

I consider it unfortunate, but the norm, to see children walking home from school gulping down a bag of barbeque potato chips and a large soda pop. However, I consider it foolish and immature to see an adult regularly consume such foods knowing that they shorten their lives. Having the "you can't teach old dogs new tricks" attitude is a sign of hopelessness, especially since the cliché applies to dogs and not humans. "As a man thinketh, so is he," is a more positive and applicable saying (scripture) in this case. Our mode of thinking not only affects our health, but it also influences our successes. If we think good health and longevity, then that is exactly what we will get. Thinking this way will lead to actions that will ensure a more healthy and prosperous life.

Many African-Americans, because of our past experiences in the United States, may be leery about new viewpoints and change. This is especially true when it is introduced by other African-Americans. The fact that you have read this book to this point indicates that you are someone open to change and a seeking a different way of life. I encourage you to explore other sources, as long as it directs you toward a healthier and longer life. The only way to do this is by checking the facts presented to you and by doing your own research. This way, your new way of thinking can be confirmed.

Positive thinking can be very challenging at times. It is important to maintain a positive look at life and sustain your healthy behaviors.

Here are a few tips:

- **Develop a plan/goal.** Making a plan to eat right and live longer is always the first step to jumpstarting a healthy life style. Preparing a healthy lunch and planning lunchtime activities is a sure way stick with it. You may want to write your goals down and read them daily, just as many of us do our Bible verses. They may be shared with others or kept private, just do it! It is also important that you start off with realistic goals but be sure not to set them too low.

- **Affiliate yourself with good role models and eliminate negative company.** Recognize and acknowledge others (friends, colleagues, family members) that display healthy habits. There is always someone around that will choose water with lemon instead of soda pop. Or, a co-worker that walks during lunch instead of chomping down the extra calories with the rest of the cafeteria. These are people you should develop "healthy" relationships with. You can learn a lot from them and you now have a lot to offer them as well. For this purpose, stay away from those who have no respect for healthy living. Once you have your system down packed, then reach out to those who need your healthy living guidance.

- **Reward yourself after each accomplishment.** Treat yourself to a nice bath, massage or something of the sort whenever you reach a short term goal (i.e. a 5 pound weight loss, no cigarettes for 7 days, no beef or pork for 30 days

- **Create support.** It is always a good idea to create a support system. You can do this by making a pact with your family and other health conscious partners. Be open and honest with yourself and others so that you all can look for signs of weakness and gently encourage and remind each other of the importance of a healthy life style. If comfortable, tell your friends and family about your new life style changes. Educate yourself in detail as you will probably be asked to explain your new life style changes. Be careful not to waste your time on educating the nay sayers.

Studies have been conducted to measure the success of positive-thinking and found that those who think they can lose weight by eating differently or increase their exercise, actually do! These people have also been found to be more successful than people with less faith in themselves. Case in point, learning how trans-fats and saturated fats destroy arteries and lead to a heart attack will force you to think twice about putting them in your body. This positive thinking will be displayed in you no longer stopping at your favorite fast food restaurant for the greasy burger and french fries. Eventually, you will no longer desire them and the thought of eating them or feeding them to your family will disgust you.

Ultimately, the inner health that we should all desire is one of peace and harmony. It is enchanting to know that Jesus said: "Peace is what I leave you; it is my own peace that I give you." (John 14:27. Good News Bible. Good News

Translation). Christ often greeted people simply by saying "peace." As most of us already know, As Salāmu `Alaykum is an Arabic language greeting used in both Muslim and Christian cultures. It means "Peace be upon you." It is also transliterated as Assalamu 'Alaikum or As-salaamu Alaikum. The traditional response is "wa `Alaykum As-Salām," meaning "and on you be peace."

Often times, a "peace of mind" is very hard to find. Life has a way of introducing situations not conducive to easy living. In other words, life can be very stressful and cause mental disarray. This can have a negative impact on marriages, job performance, parenting and of course, one's health. These things can also cause stress and disrupt your mental harmony. Old African thinking is that stress can lead to illnesses of all sorts as well as death. As a matter of scientific fact, stress lowers the immune system. A lowered immune system means that your body is weak and cannot fight off disease (infections, cancers, inflammation, heart attacks, etc.).

Since stress is a major cause of unhappiness among humans, we must have ways to cope with it. First, try to identify the things in your life that prevent your joy. It could be your weight, marriage, conflict at work, a recent death or illness within your family, etc. Once you identify and begin to understand the stressor, you can better figure out a way to deal with or eliminate it. Consider its duration, strength and its effect on your body.

Because chronic stress can be associated with other mental conditions such as depression or anxiety, seek immediate professional help if you experience any of the following:

- Prolonged feelings of sadness or worthlessness
- Suicidal thoughts
- Homicidal thoughts
- Difficulty sleeping
- Panic attacks
- Change in appetite
- Muscle tenderness or soreness
- Frequent headaches
- Gastrointestinal problems
- Abuse alcohol or drugs

We have got to remember that we have the ability to help our bodies by using our minds. *God hath not given us the spirit of fear; but of power, and of love, and of a sound mind* (2 Timothy 1:7, King James Version). Even scientists are accepting the fact that the brain functions in creating thoughts and feelings and through this knowledge we are now gaining tools that assist us in bringing about healing to our physical and emotional ailments. The prognosis is always good when the final state is psychological freedom and spiritual harmony. As a Christian, this practice is not new and "scientific discovery" only makes Paul's admonition in Romans 12:1 a reality: *"And be not conformed to this world: but be ye transformed by the renewing of your mind, that ye may prove what is that good, and acceptable, and perfect, will of God."*

When needed, African-Americans must turn to support groups and stress relief activities such as exercise and meditation. These, and many other mind strengthening behaviors, build up the immune system by altering stress hormone levels.

4. Change your level of activity.

"Physical exercise has some value, but spiritual exercise is value in every way..." (1Timothy 4:8. Good News Bible, Good News translation).

Notice that this biblical verse does not say that exercise has no value, because it does. In fact, the National institute of Health says that exercise can help one lose weight, lower cholesterol levels, reduce chances of getting diabetes and lower blood pressure. All four of which greatly and disproportionately affect the African-American community. Quite frankly, exercise is the ultimate anti-aging agent.

Exercise can reverse depression and provides an increase in self esteem. Unfortunately, those who suffer from depression and worthlessness are the least likely to began an exercise program of any type. These traits also lead to increased appetites, obesity as well as other illnesses.

Exercise, like eating right, usually requires a significant lifestyle change and sacrifice. People come up with a variety of excuses as to why they cannot exercise regularly. Something as simple as walking your dog or taking a walk during lunch each day lends to a healthier life.

5. **Educate your family and friends on proper eating and the importance of exercise.**

"Thoughtless words can wound as deeply as any sword, but wisely spoken words can heal." (Proverbs 12:18. Good News Bible, Good News Translation)

In December 2006, I visited 3 different book stores taking advantage of their 40% off coupons. It disappointed me dearly that I found only a few other African-Americans in one store and none in the other two. Forty percent off of any book, I would think, would be attractive to more than two African-Americans in the Detroit Metropolitan area. Certainly, a 40% off sale on clothing or unhealthy foods would get us out in droves. Maybe this was the point many tried to make to me when they advised that I not write a book specifically for African-Americans for fear that it would be read. You, on the other hand, are unlike the "stereotypical black" that we often hear and read about or who these nay sayers warned me of. I thank you dearly for beginning (or continuing) your health journey with this book, but your responsibility doesn't stop here. How to eat and live longer must be shared with the rest of our community. Start by informing your friends and family on what you have learned about the devil's trickery as it relates to the foods we eat.

African-Americans, not the U.S government or the medical arena, must rid ourselves of the illogical rationalities and health care disparities that have been slaughtering our parents, grandparents, children and grandchildren for hundreds of years.

The first place to start is with "self." Realizing that your body is a temple...owned by God and made for the edification of God. You must learn the "do's" and "don'ts" of eating, adopt an exercise program and then master them both to the best of your ability.

Next, you have to extend this knowledge to your family members, regardless of their age. The younger the family member learns, the longer your kin will begin to live. Be creative with your family to make the transition more attractive to everyone. For instance, allow every Saturday to be family exercise day. Your family should then extend such ideas to your church members, neighbors and extended family. This can be done via emails or referrals to websites, church and neighborhood health awareness programs and simple conversations in public places. Challenge your block club presidents, fraternity & sorority presidents, Pastors and community leaders to reach their ideal body weights and stay there. Regardless of how we decide to do it, it must be done!

6. **Maintain this new way of life.**

"My dear friend, I pray that everything may go well with you and that you may be in good health, as I know you are well in spirit." (3 John 1:2-3. Good News Bible, Good News Translation).

This is not a fly-by-night doctrine or a yo-yo diet with healthy commendations...this is a way of life! We must forever love and respect ourselves enough to seek prosperity and longevity as it relates to our existence. We were created as a people of great esteem and served as the epitome of excellence for the rest of the world. Our mental, physical and spiritual realms were far removed from any other group of persons. God, who makes no mistakes, created our bodies after His own image which is perfection. Our impious way of life made us imperfect and the wages of such actions are sickness and early death.

To others, we are a loving, kind and caring people. To ourselves, we are unknowingly hateful, apathetic and unfair. The book of Mathew (19:19) tells us that we are to love our neighbors as ourselves. The question now becomes: Do we love ourselves? The time has come for African-Americans to reclaim our position as people of dignity, deserving respect and of wholesome ways. We must respect our minds by building its monuments of intelligence and display our love of God's temples by eating foods that help (not harm) us.

In order to not suffer from the sicknesses that other African-Americans experience, you must be different. And being different means to do things dissimilar, including the way you think, eat and maintain your new and improved way of doing things. No longer eating like the rest of your friends and family sets you apart from them and in this sense, this is good. Just as it was necessary for Jesus to be in the world *but not of the world*, so should you! You will find initially that people will challenge and criticize you but eventually your discipline will spark their interest. Others will notice the youthfulness of your skin, your increased energy level and weight loss (if needed). Your continued restraint from that unhealthy life style will perfect your character and generate persistence. Also, since we reap what we sow; the more persistent we are in sowing, the more we will eventually reap. So be sure to sow seeds of knowledge, health and longevity.

With this in mind and in action, no longer shall my people perish because of the lack of knowledge.

References

Introduction

1)   *Morbid obesity in toddlers linked to lower IQ.* (Friday, September 7, 2006). [Online]. Available: www.cbc.ca./health/story/2006/09/01/obesity-iq.html.

Chapter 1

1)   *Secrets of the dead. Case file: Search for the first human being.* (November, 2004). [Online]. Available: www.pbs.org/wnet/secrets/case_firsthuman/.

Chapter 4

1)   *Gullah Pride.* [Online]. Available: www.geocities.com/gullahpride/

2)   *Saving Gullah.* (2003). The State Newspaper. Sunday, September 28, 2003. Page 4.

Chapter 5

1)   *Milk.* [Online]. Available: www.wordnet-online.com.

2)   *Boning up on Calcium and Osteoporosis.* [Online]. Available: www.pcrm.org/health/veginfo/nutritionfaq.html C

3)   Feskanich D et al. (1997). *Milk, Dietary Calcium, and Bone Fractures in Women: a 12-year prospective study.* The American Journal of Public health. 87 (6) 992-7.

4)   Deardorff, Julie. *Not Milk?* New research questions value – if not safety of dairy. Chicago Tribune. (2006).   [Online].   Available: **www.chicagotribune.com**. (2006).

Chapter 7

1)   Colbert, Don. July 2005. *What would Jesus Eat?* Nelson Books.

2)   *USDA Economic Research Service. (2005). Cattle and Beef.* [Online]. ERSLDPM13502. 25pp. Available: **www.ers.usda.gov**. October 7, 2005.

3)   Howenstine, James. (2004). *High meat intake appears to cause cancer and heart attacks.* [Online]. Available: **www.newswithviews.com**. (December 2004).

4)   *Beef.* Edutainment. Boogie Down Productions. (July 17, 1990).

Chapter 10

1)   Information about caffeine Dependence. Caffeine and Health. (2003). [Online]. Available: **www.caffeinedependence.org/caffeine_depende nce.html**. (2003).

2)   *Liquid Candy. How soft drinks are harming America's health.* Center for Science in the public interest. [Online].   Available: **www.cspinet.org/liquidcandy/**.

Chapter 12

1) The Worst Mistake In The History Of The Human Race.)May 1987. Pp 64-66). [Online]. Available: http://anthropology.lbcc.edu/handoutsdocs/mis take.pdf.

Chapter 14

1) Holton, Noel. (2004). *African-Americans and Hypertension: A Q&A with UM Cardiologist Elijah Saunders.* [Online]. Available: **www.umm.edu/heart/blood_pressure.html**.

2) Flack MD, John M, Peters MSN, Rosalind M. (October 1, 2000). *Salt Sensitivity and Hypertension in African-Americans: Implications for Cardiovascular Disease. Prog Cariovasc Nurs* 15 (4): 138-144, 2000. Le Jacq Communications, Inc.

3) Jacobson Ph D, Michael F. (2005). Salt: The forgotten Killer and FDA's failure to protect the public's health. Center for Science in the Public Interest. [Online]. Available: **http://cspinet.org/salt/saltreport.pdf**. (2005).

Chapter 15

1) Black vegetarians. (2003). [Online]. Available: **www.blackvegetarians.org**

2) Pfeil, Ricky. (2001). *Kingdom Keys Network.* [Online]. Available: **www.kingdomkeys.org/ricky**.

3) Barbara, David. Day, Sherri. (June 20, 2003). *McDonalds' seeking cut in antibiotics in its meat.* The New York Times. (March 28, 2007). [Online]. Available: **http://query.nytimes.com/gst/fullpage.html**

341

Chapter 17

1)   Torgan ph D, Carol (June 2003). Childhood
        Obesity on the Rise. The NIH: Word on Health.
        [ONLINE].   Available:
        http://www.nih/gov/news/wordonhealth/june
        2002/childhoodobesity.htm.(2002).

Chapter 18

1)   *Dietary Goals for the United States: Statement of*
        Senator George McGovern on the publication goals for
        the United States. (January 14, 1977). [Online].
        Available:
        www.anaturalway.com/dietary_goals3.html

Chapter 19

1)   Flack MD, John M, Peters MSN, Rosalind M.
        (October 1, 2000). *Salt Sensitivity and Hypertension*
        in African-Americans: Implications for Cardiovascular
        Disease. Prog Cariovasc Nurs 15 (4): 138-144, 2000.
        Le Jacq Communications, Inc.

Chapter 20

1)   Martin, Wayne. (August – September 2005).
        Vegetarian diet for arthritis. Townsend letter for the
        Doctors and patients. (2005). The Townsend letter
        Group.

Chapter 22

1)   Clark, Carol. (2001). Blueprint of the body: On the
        threshold of a brave new world. [Online].
        Available:
        http://www.cnn.com/specials/2000/genome/story/
        overview

Chapter 25

1)   Easton, John. (December 2, 1999). *Lack of Sleep Alters Hormones, Metabolism*. (Vol. 19 No. 6). The University of Chicago Chronicle. [Online]. Available: http://chronicle.uchicago.edu/991202/sleep.shtml. (1999).

2-3)   *Too little sleep combined with holiday overeating may increase risk of obesity.* (2007). [Online]. Available: www.sleepfoundation.org. (November 18, 2004).

Chapter 26

1)   *George Washington Carver Quotes.* [Online]. Available: http://en.thinkexist.com/quotation/reading_about _nature_is_fine_but_if_a_person/207960.html

Chapter 28

1)   Digital Hippocrates; Book I. (1971/ Replication of 1935 edition). [Online]. Available: www.chit.org/sandbox/dh/celsusenglish/page.2 1.a.php-5k

Chapter 29

1)   *Fasting and Detox.* (March 8, 2007). [Online]. Available: http://www/astangayogasurrey.com

Chapter 32

1)   *Life, and How We Live It.* [Online]. Available: http://littlecalamity.tripod.com/poetry/life.html